TESTIMONIES FROM REAL PEOPLE LIKE YOU FOR
BUNS OF STEEL®

"Actually, I've seen amazing results. I feel more comfortable walking around in a bathing suit. I am not as self-conscious, I don't run to throw a towel or shirt on."
—Allison Beck

"I was a size 12 and went down to a 7."
—Elaine Brown

"I really found I could see results right away. I used the tapes for a week and noticed the results in my legs immediately. I felt like my legs were really toned . . . I always felt like I had a good workout."
—Candace Dale

"My whole family has been blessed with the love handles. With BUNS OF STEEL®, mine have been vanishing on a daily basis. Great results!"
—Lisa Coccodrille

"I lost 22 pounds! I have a lot more energy and I feel amazing."
—Susie Kurtz

"Nothing has made my self-esteem soar more than using the BUNS OF STEEL® exercise tapes. They make me feel wonderful!"
—Kathleen Naccarato-McFadden

"I gained 57 pounds during my pregnancy. I started doing BUNS OF STEEL® along with a low-fat diet and the weight just kept coming off. Nine months later, the roll on my tummy was gone and my thighs no longer rub when I walk. Thanks to BUNS OF STEEL®, I look and feel great!"
—Marianthe Gavalas

ENDORSEMENTS FROM EXPERTS AND THE PRESS FOR THE
BUNS OF STEEL® VIDEOTAPES

"The best aerobics and toning tapes I've seen."
—Jeannine Crouse, fitness instructor

"On a rating scale of one to four stars, I award the BUNS OF STEEL PLATINUM series four stars and I highly recommend it."
—Anne Cartwright, exercise physiologist

more . . .

"The exercises are low-impact which helps avoid stress on the joints of the body, and the aerobics are an excellent way to lose weight."
—Jeffrey Dermksian, M.D., orthopedic surgeon

"From beginning to end and top to bottom, this book is the textbook of toning for today's fitness consumer!"
—Leslie Scott, executive director, The Health Instructor Network

"You may smile at the results . . . Impressive."
—*New Body*

"Short and simple. Loved the cool-down!"
—*San Francisco Chronicle*

"[Nancy Kerrigan] . . . adapted part of her training regimen to the *Abs of Steel*® workout video."
—*USA Today*

"People laughed at the titles when these target-training tapes came out, but dedicated users of the specialized videos have the last laugh when they don their trendy thongs and skintight exercise togs . . . anyone who performs these intensive tapes regularly cannot help but tighten their buns. . . . These tapes have become classics for shaping specific problem areas."
—*Your Health*

Buns of Steel® Total-Body Workout

Leisa Hart and Liz Neporent, M.A.

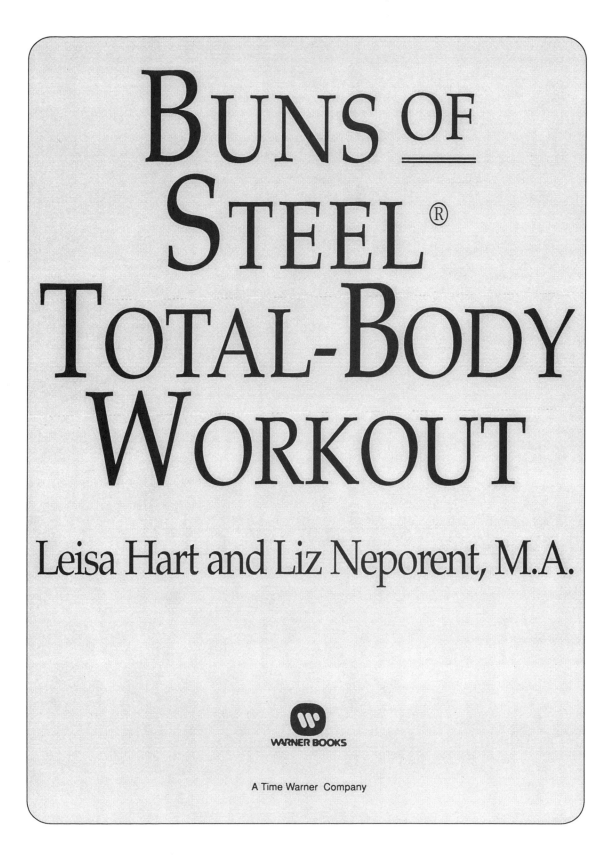

WARNER BOOKS

A Time Warner Company

Neither the program in this book, nor any other exercise program, should be followed without first consulting a health care professional. If you have any special conditions requiring attention, you should consult with your health care professional regularly regarding possible modification of the program contained in this book.

Warner Books, Inc., 1271 Avenue of the Americas, New York, NY 10020

Ⓦ A Time Warner Company

Printed in the United States of America

ISBN 0-446-67089-8

Book design by Giorgetta Bell McRee
Cover design by Mike Stromberg
Cover and interior photographs by Don Banks

Acknowledgments

Leisa—

To Momma and Daddy. Thank you for giving me my confidence. With your love I feel I can accomplish anything.

To my niece, Tiffany Bolfing, Texas A&M's Buns of Steel. Study Hard! You have so much potential.

To my beautiful sister Barbie Wicker. Thanks for believing in me—I want to be just like you when I grow up.

Thanks to the entire Bolfing family. Each of you in your own special way has helped me to become what I am today.

To Howard Maier. Thank you for the chance of a lifetime—here's to success!

To Melissa Berman of The Maier Group. Your constant professionalism has made my job easier and your compassion has made me feel right at home with The Maier Group.

To Liz Neporent. Your unwavering dedication to fitness has inspired me to give 110 percent.

To Tom Eades, my best bud and number one fan. Thanks for believing in me.

To my two favorite mentors, Leslie Scott of the Health Instructors Network and Terri Arends of the Premier Athletic Club. Your brilliance in your fields has helped me to grow.

To David Gray, my video man. Thanks for making me look so good—I couldn't have done it without you!

Liz—

To Mom and Dad, Granny, Mark, Lori, Richie, Jill, and Ted. Thanks for *everything*.

To everyone at Frontline Fitness, especially Norman Zinker, Craig Marson, Holly Byrne, Bob Welter, Terry Certain, and Vincent Metzo. Thanks for your patience, hard work, and expertise.

Thanks to Howard Maier and everyone else at The Maier Group, especially the very sane Melissa Berman.

To Leisa Hart. Thanks for your professionalism, talent, intelligence, and great buns!

Thanks to everyone at Goldman Sachs and Salomon Brothers, especially Bob Katz, Arline Mann, and Ellen and Bill Kealy.

Thanks to Richard Miller of the Gym Source for his friendship and belief in me from the start.

To my professors Emily Wugholter, James Santomier, Patty Hogan, and Gil Gleim. Thanks for being such great teachers.

Thanks to Eli Jacobson, the world's foremost expert on exercise and tax law.

To Cecele Fraenkle. Thanks for your consistently good advice and your belief in me.

To Mary Duffy, Peg Moline, Margaret Pierpont, and all my other terrific magazine editors. Thanks for giving me a break when I needed one, and for all your advice, support, and friendship.

Finally to my husband, Jay Shafran. Thanks for believing in me and for helping me believe in myself.

Contents

PART II

Foreword

Buns of Steel has become the exercise video phenomenon of the 1990s. As president of the company that owns *Buns of Steel*, I am often given the credit for its creation. Yet the success of this video is due to many people. I didn't invent *Buns of Steel*. Greg Smithey, an aerobics instructor, who at the time lived in Alaska, did. He created the first *Buns of Steel* video, and licensed it to Lee Spieker of Fit Video. In 1988 Fit Video licensed the video to The Maier Group. Later, Greg licensed all rights to *Buns of Steel* to The Maier Group, which has enabled us to develop this breakthrough phenomenon.

Initially, *Buns of Steel* sales were relatively slow because no one knew about the video. But over the past few years sales have skyrocketed as word-of-mouth recommendations and our advertising created awareness among exercise enthusiasts. The Buns of Steel series now has a market share of approximately 50 percent of all the exercise videos sold, and today the workouts include *Abs of Steel, Legs of Steel, Thighs of Steel,* and even a *Pregnancy Workout.* Our Platinum series, which is featured in our successful infomercials, adds aerobics to the toning exercises *Buns of Steel* is known for. Recently, we have introduced a new Men of Steel series and the Buns of Steel Mind/Body series, including Yoga and Tai-Chi.

Through the years we've been blessed with talented fitness instructors who provide exercises that work. All of our instructors are professional fitness experts who are truly dedicated to good, safe, effective, motivating workouts. I would like to thank Tamilee Webb, Marsha Macro, Lynne Brick, Tracy York, Donna Richardson, Madeleine Lewis, Leisa Hart, Gilad Janklowicz, Kurt Brungardt, Marguerite Baca, and Dominic Stephano who have all led *Buns of Steel* programs. Talented producers like Andrea Ambandos and Lee Spieker have produced our videos and I thank them. Steve Kaplan and Geraldine Newman bring *Buns of Steel* to life in our television commercials.

That *Buns of Steel* ''look'' in our packaging and magazine advertising is primarily the work of Milt Polowski and David DiNuccio. Milt is also largely responsible for the great look of this book. I thank the authors, Leisa Hart and Liz Neporent, and all the individuals from Warner Books and The Maier Group who have contributed their efforts to making this book.

Since this is the first *Buns of Steel* book, let me take a moment to thank all Maier Groupers for all their efforts in bringing Buns of Steel programs to the public: Ellen Hochman, Gene Moriarty, Tom Morton, Candy Barth, Melissa Berman, Joan Cox, and all the others.

I would also like to thank my wife, Margaret Cuomo Maier, for bringing such joy to me, and to my children, Melissa, Pablo and Lindsay, who have all been such an important part of my life.

Buns of Steel is a commitment for The Maier Group to bring excellent fitness to everyone's life. Enjoy.

—HOWARD S. MAIER

Introduction

A reputation for combining the latest exercise routines with the most effective body-shaping techniques has made the Buns of Steel exercise videos number one best-sellers. They're recognized by consumers and fitness experts alike as the best muscle toning workouts on the market. So why a Buns of Steel book? The *Buns of Steel Total-Body Workout* book takes the Buns of Steel concept one step farther. It's like having the entire video collection at your fingertips. Not only is it a state-of-the-art, highly effective, results-oriented program, it also contains invaluable tips on how to individualize each and every exercise routine to meet your needs. And there's lots of information on how to keep things fresh and interesting—so you can always create an entirely new workout, something not possible with videos.

Another advantage the *Buns of Steel Total-Body Workout* has over an exercise video: You can take it with you wherever you go. All you need is this book and some good old-fashioned muscle power—and you can quickly turn your desire for tighter buns, trimmer thighs, and a flatter stomach into reality anywhere, anytime. Here's still more good news. As you improve, the *Buns of Steel Total-Body Workout* adapts right along with you. The program we've laid out for you in the chapters to follow gives you plenty of choices. Rather than getting one workout, as you do with an exercise video, we'll show you how to modify each exercise and how to fine-tune your program to suit your needs, preferences, and improving fitness level. All this variety will add a spark of excitement to your exercise routine—a spark that will burst into flame once you see and feel the results!

Any way you use it, the program in this book has been expertly designed so you'll see improvements fast. Your body will respond immediately, and you'll look better than you ever dreamed possible.

It's a fact: Your body is genetically destined to lose or gain weight in a particular pattern. Take a look at your mother, your grandmother, or some other close female relatives. Chances are, if they have "thunder thighs" or "hanging triceps," so will you. After all, you can't fight genetics, right? Wrong! We'll show you that you *can* break the mold! The way to remold your body is not through stringent dieting. Even if you lose twenty pounds, you may be left with a smaller version of the same proportions. Fortunately there *is* a way you can take aim at your trouble zones and make specific changes in your body exactly where you want them. We call it *target toning*.

What is target toning? It's a method that zeroes in on an exact area of your body and improves it through the use of resistance and precise, focused movements. Resistance refers to the amount of work you give your muscles. In this program you'll add resistance in the form of dumbbells, ankle weights, exercise bands, or simply the weight of your own body. This resistance places tension on your muscles and stimulates them to work harder. The result: you'll firm, tighten, and tone. At the same time, you'll lose inches of fat. You'll also be carving sexy curves of muscle into your body. Best of all, your metamorphosis will begin with your very first Buns of Steel workout.

With target toning, you don't need to do more than fifteen repetitions of an exercise. When you can do those fifteen repetitions easily, you make the move more challenging by adding resistance or changing the intensity of the exercise. You're always pushing yourself toward your potential—and toward your ultimate toning goals. Doing fewer, more concentrated reps means you can target tone your buns, or any other part of your body, in as little as ten minutes a day. You'll see significant changes after just a few weeks without having to dedicate your entire life to your workout regimen. Target toning is *fast*, and it really works.

But the real secret to the Buns of Steel method? *The most effective target toning exercises you'll ever do.* Each move is designed to work deep into your target muscle and change its shape. You won't waste time because we've selected only exercises that we know will pay off. From the very first repetition you'll feel every exercise, in every routine, exactly where you should. And it won't be long before you *see* tangible evidence of your efforts.

Now that you have a good understanding of why the *Buns of Steel Total-Body Workout* is such an effective program and why it works so much better than any other body reshaping method, let's get started! Here's what's going to take place over the next few weeks:

As you read through the following chapters and begin to do the target toning routines, you'll feel your enthusiasm and excitement build. You'll quickly realize that if shapelier buns, flatter abs, firmer hips and thighs, and a sculpted upper body are your aims, then doing the *Buns of Steel Total-Body Workout* has put you on the right track.

In just a few short weeks of target toning you'll see and feel your body molding itself into something special, something it's never been before. Your muscles will be tighter and more defined, and a considerable amount of fat will melt away from your body. You'll see a hard, sexy physique begin to take shape. You'll be stronger, stand up straighter, and have more energy than you've had in years. Even if you dreaded exercising in the past, you'll look forward eagerly to each target toning session because you know you're looking better and better.

So if you've been searching for a workout program that really delivers, picking up this book is the best thing you've ever done. Sound good? Then get ready to create the body you've always wanted with the *Buns of Steel Total-Body Workout!*

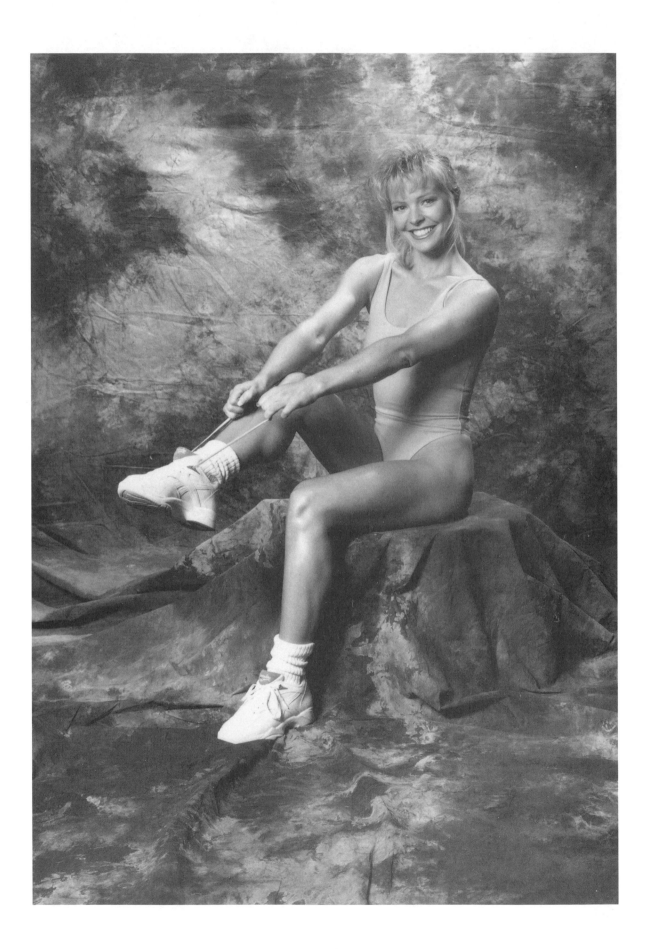

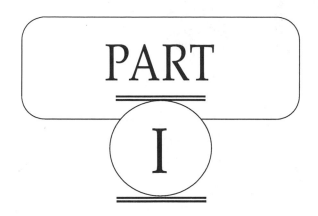

PART

I

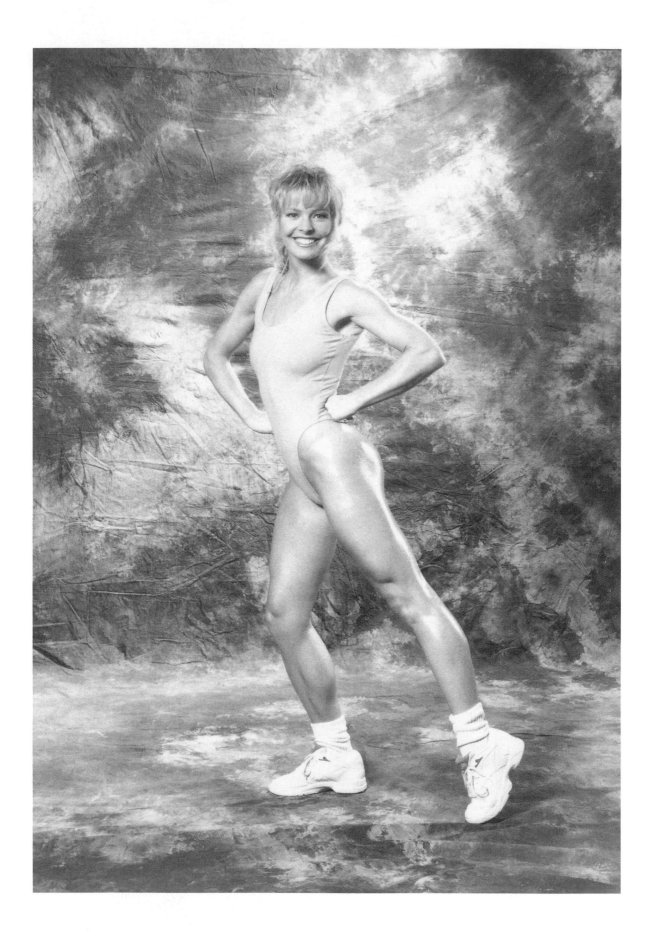

The Buns of Steel Philosophy

Train hard, train consistently, train smart. That's the Buns of Steel philosophy. Our training program sends you down the most direct path toward success because it adheres to these three principles. No other body-shaping method can promise you the results you'll get from this program, pay such close attention to injury prevention, and still keep things fresh and exciting. That's why, whether your target toning goal is firmer buns, trimmer thighs, or a tighter tummy, the Total-Body Workout can help you meet, even exceed, your expectations.

Some people just want to tone what they've got, while others are looking to do a whole body makeover. Whatever your target toning goals are, you can achieve them by exercising with this program. These workouts are focused to yield *results*. You really *will* tighten your entire body and squeeze out fat if you faithfully do the exercise routines in this book. It's that simple.

However, the pace of the results depends upon several factors: your current physical condition, your age, your metabolism, your genetics, and, of course, the exercise program you choose. Since we don't waste any space or any of your energy on anything that isn't effective, *everyone* who follows the Buns of Steel program will see results. How long will it take? You'll probably begin to see noticeable improvements in most areas of your body in about one month. In roughly eight weeks' time prepare yourself for the deluge of compliments you'll receive on your new, slimmer, sleeker, shapelier body!

What's Your Type?

As we've said, the word *results* means different things to different people. And, while there's no doubt you can improve your appearance by doing our workouts, we think it's important to have realistic expectations. If you're five feet two and curvy, you can't expect a six-foot-tall fashion model's body to emerge after a few weeks of training.

Trying to achieve a look that doesn't mesh with your body type is counter-productive. Playing up your natural assets is much more rewarding. Exactly what type of body do you have, and how will it respond to training?

Essentially, the way a woman is shaped falls into one of three broad categories: endomorph, ectomorph, or mesomorph. It's simply a matter of determining what your body type is in order to realize your possibilities. Like most women, you probably have some characteristics of all three body types, but overall you resemble one type most:

Endomorphs have round, smooth bodies and large bones. Their hips are wider than their shoulders, and their weight is concentrated below the waist. When in shape, endomorphs possess both curves and cuts (muscle definition), not to mention tremendous sex appeal. Target toning makes endomorphs look muscular yet beautifully feminine.

Since endomorphs tend to hold on to body fat a bit more than other body types, target toning is the perfect solution to shaping up any trouble zones. It adds muscle to create a balance between the upper and lower body and speeds up the metabolism so the body burns fat more quickly. By doing the Buns of Steel program, endomorphs can look forward to a firmly toned body with the curvy sensuality of a big-screen star.

If you're an **ectomorph,** you're slender with shoulders and hips that are approximately the same width. You have a small to medium frame and tend toward an angular look. Other body types envy your ability to repel excess body fat, but your body may also have resisted the development of lean muscle tissue up till now. Training with the *Buns of Steel Total-Body Workout* will help you add shape, proportion, and definition to your physique. Start with a straight, skinny body, add a few weeks of target toning, and presto! The ectomorph can carve sexy, shapely curves into her lean frame. That's the way it goes with ectomorphs: you may start out thin and lanky, but you'll end up looking firm, muscular, and curvaceous.

The **mesomorph** is the most "athletic" looking of the three body types. She has a muscular, rectangular outline with strong bones and broad shoulders. Her weight is distributed more or less evenly, and her hips are usually not quite as wide as her shoulders. If you're a mesomorph, you'll be pleased how quickly you can fine-tune your body's natural athleticism. Mesomorphs seem to soak up the benefits of target toning exercises the way a sponge soaks up water! Adding muscle while chiseling away body fat will reveal firm yet feminine proportions. Out-of-shape mesomorphs tend to be stocky but not fat. Yet even before they start exercising, their symmetrically perfect proportions are obvious. For mesomorphs a little target toning truly does go a long way!

TYPECASTING

Like most people, you're probably a combination of body types. Though your appearance will change as you lose fat and gain muscle, your basic shape is determined by your genetics. Take the test below to determine which of the three basic body types you most closely resemble. You'll need a mirror, a tape measure, and about fifteen minutes. Choose the most appropriate answer to each question:

1. Encircle your wrist, using your middle finger and thumb. They
    a. don't touch.
    b. just touch.
    c. touch with some overlapping.

2. Bend your elbow and make a muscle by tightening your fist. With your other hand, find the bulge of your upper arm that begins near the crease above your elbow. Using the width of your fingers, measure the distance between the start of this bulge and the crease in your arm. This distance is

    a. one finger's width.

    b. two fingers' width.

    c. three fingers' width or more.

3. Stand sideways next to a mirror. Balance yourself on one leg, standing as much on tiptoe as you can without falling over. Note the point at which the bulge of your calf muscle stops closest to your heel. Come down from tiptoe and look at where this point is in relation to the distance between the back of your heel and the back of your knee. Your calf muscle covers

    a. about three-quarters of the distance between the back of the knee and the heel.

    b. about half the distance between the back of the knee and the heel.

    c. about one-quarter of the distance between the back of the knee and the heel.

4. Measure your hips and waist. Subtract your waist from your hip measurement. The difference is

    a. less than two inches.

    b. more than two but less than eight inches.

    c. eight inches or more.

5. With your arm hanging at your side, measure the largest part of your upper arm. Flex your arm (as you did in question 2) and measure at the same point. Subtract the hanging measurement from the flexed measurement. The difference between them is

    a. less than one-quarter of an inch.

    b. between one-quarter of an inch and one inch.

    c. greater than one inch.

6. Stand in front of a mirror and assess your body.

    a. It is rounded, especially at the hips, elbows, and knees. Your hips are wider than your shoulders. Most of your weight is concentrated in the hips and thighs.

    b. It has a muscular, "rectangular" outline. Your shoulders are wider than your hips. Your weight is distributed more or less evenly between the upper and lower body.

    c. It is sharp and angular, especially the elbows, hips, and knees. Your shoulders and hips are approximately the same width.

7. You are
- a. overweight.
- b. average weight.
- c. below average weight.

If you have three or more (a.) answers, your body type is closest to endomorph. If you chose three or more (b.) answers, your body type is closest to mesomorph. If you chose three or more (c.) answers, your body is closest to ectomorph. If your answers were more or less evenly spread between two body types, consider yourself a true combination body type such as a meso-endomorph.

Get Motivated with the S.O.L.I.D. Approach

Let's face it, motivation is all about having a positive attitude. If you feel good about what you're doing, it takes no effort to keep doing it. Of course, maintaining a positive attitude can be linked directly to results. When you see your buns reshaping or definition beginning to form around your middle, you can't help but look forward to your next workout. That's the beauty of target toning: the more you do it, the better you look.

But how do you know you're getting results? We think it's important to have a consistent, scientific method of measuring progress. Sure you'll see a change when you look in the mirror, but to generate excitement and keep you psyched, there's nothing like hard evidence that your target toning routine is working. We've developed the S.O.L.I.D. method of results measurement so you can quantify your progress by defining your expectations.

Before you begin your target toning program, carefully read through each point of the S.O.L.I.D. system. Grab a piece of paper and a pen. Write down some notes on each item, and put these notes up on your refrigerator or on your bathroom mirror so you can refer to them from time to time. In about a month look back at where you started and see how far you've come. See if that doesn't help your motivation (not to mention your self-esteem) soar!

Starting point. Where are you beginning? One of the quickest, most reliable ways to determine this is by taking body measurements. Get a measuring tape and take each measurement to the nearest quarter inch. Here are the areas you should measure: the widest part of your upper and lower leg, around your hips and buns, the smallest part of your waist, your chest over the center of your breasts, and the largest circumference of your upper arm when your elbow is completely straightened. Get your piece of paper and write down each measurement and the date you took it. Now do your Buns of Steel Total-Body Workout faithfully for a month. Remeasure. There's proof positive of your success in the form of lost inches!

Objectives. Do you want a smaller waist? Better buns? Write your goals down and keep them in mind as you go through your workouts. Make your objectives as detailed and specific as you can. For instance, rather than simply saying you want to lose weight, determine your present body fat (a more accurate measure of fitness and appearance) and then aim to drop a specific and *realistic* number of percentage points. Allow yourself some time to achieve these goals. Remember, Rome wasn't built in a day, so give yourself permission not to race to reshape your body!

Layout. Lay out a plan to get from point A (your starting point) to point B (your goals). We've taken care of that for you with the effective routines you'll find at the end of every exercise chapter. Still, it helps to keep in mind a general plan of attack. Example: Are you going to do the ten-, fifteen-, or twenty-minute routines at the end of each chapter? Are you going to devote more time to working on your abs or your buns? Will you work out in the morning or the evening? Write down a few sentences describing your game plan. Your program will work and you'll stay motivated because you'll start with your goals in mind and work toward them in a sensible, systematic manner.

Individualize. Again, we've taken care of that for you. We've given you the ability to make each exercise easier or harder so you get the exact amount of training you need. Take some time to think about how you can best fit your target toning sessions into your day. Jot down important considerations such as time constraints, travel plans, other obligations, then choose the customized routines that best match your life-style. The more you adapt the Total-Body Workout to your needs, the more likely you are to stick with it.

Diary. Keeping an exercise diary is a terrific motivator. It's tangible proof that you're working toward your goals. Go ahead and detail your workouts on your piece of paper for a month. When you run out of room, you may want to purchase a commercial exercise log or a book with blank pages to help you keep track of your information on a more permanent basis.

Some important details you should record: the date you worked out; the name of the exercises or routine, number of sets and repetitions, and order of exercises you performed; how long your target toning session took to complete; the difficulty of your workout on a scale of one to five. Make notes of things you need to change when you do your next workout, such as the amount of weight or the particular version of an exercise.

A MEASUREMENT WITH MUSCLE

In the weeks ahead, your body weight may stay more or less the same, even though you drop a dress size or find that you're able to wear a pair of jeans you haven't fit into in years. The reason: Since muscle is denser than fat, it takes up less room but weighs more per square inch. In fact, one pound of fat takes up three times as much space as a pound of muscle.

More important than how much you weigh is how much of your weight is fat and how much is lean muscle. In other words, what is your percentage of body fat? Even if the needle on your scale doesn't budge right away, target toning helps decrease your body fat percentage while adding healthy, sexy muscle. Here's a simple method of measuring body fat:

1. Measure your height in inches to the nearest inch. Mark it on the "height" line on the chart on page 13.

2. Measure your hips around the widest girth to the nearest inch. Mark it on the "hip girth" line.

3. With a ruler, draw a diagonal line from your height mark to your hip girth mark. Your body fat percentage is indicated where your line crosses the percent fat column. An ideal body fat percentage for a woman is between 16 and 26 percent. Don't obsess over this number. Use it as a starting point to get yourself moving in the right direction and then remeasure in about four to eight weeks.

Safety First

You can be confident that the exercises in this program are carefully designed to help you avoid injury. We've taken great pains to describe proper form and explain exactly how each exercise should feel when you're doing it right. If you follow our directions conscientiously and warm up and cool down properly, it's likely that you'll never have to interrupt your training because of an injury. However, there are a few safety-related details that bear mentioning at this point.

• Most injuries are the result of carelessness. Listen to your body. If you're performing a move incorrectly or using sloppy form, your body will let you know. Do a thorough reading of the exercise descriptions and follow them to the letter. We'll give you constant reminders to use good form throughout. (Also, see "Focus on Form," page 11.) Look for cues like "Keep your wrist in line with your forearm" and "Maintain a natural arch in your spine."

• Never do any exercise so quickly that your movements are abrupt or jerky. The object is to feel the exercise working your muscles, *not* your bones. We'll give you plenty of safety cues in the coming exercise chapters to remind you to move slowly through the exercises at a steady, even pace. Pay attention to directions like "Don't lock your elbows" and "Keep your knees soft."

• As you go through the Total-Body Workout you'll feel your muscles working hard and pushing past old limits. Although we don't subscribe to the "No pain, no gain" theory, you might want to think of this muscular effort as a mild *good pain*. Once you get used to feeling this "good pain," you'll come to enjoy it and understand it as your body's response to the demands target toning places upon it.

You should *never* experience what we refer to as *bad pain* while doing one of our target toning routines. Bad pain is the kind you feel in your joints rather than in your muscles; it manifests itself in the form of an aching knee, sore elbow, or tender lower back. It's important that you learn to differentiate between good pain and bad pain so you know when to work through your discomfort and when it's better to back off. Each exercise has a "Mind/Body Focus" section that explains what the exercise should feel like.

• If, in spite of everything, you do injure yourself, it's best to rest rather than continue exercising. Better to lay off completely for one week than do further damage and be forced to lay off for an even longer period of time. If possible, work around an injury by focusing your energies on the areas of your body that aren't affected by it.

FOCUS ON FORM

Your mother was right. Good posture is an instant way to appear thinner and more attractive. It's also important in terms of protecting your joints from injury—your lower back in particular. In the coming chapters you'll get continual reminders to stand up straight and practice good posture. As you target tone, keep this head-to-toe posture guide in mind:

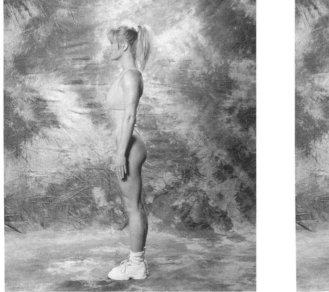 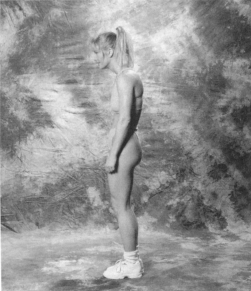

• Don't allow your head to drop forward. Keep it back in the center of your shoulders and in line with the rest of your spine.

• Relax your shoulders backward and downward.

• Keep your chest and rib cage lifted. Proper shoulder alignment will allow you to "open up" your chest.

• Stand or sit up tall and maintain a natural arch in your spine.

• Pull your abdominals in toward your spine.

• When you stand, your legs should be straight, but don't "lock" your knees (this will cause your lower back to overarch). Your weight should be distributed evenly between both feet. When you are seated, your knees should be comfortably bent with your feet flat on the floor.

Hurts So Good

Some muscle soreness is a normal consequence of proper training, at least initially. You should feel a pleasant sort of muscle fatigue after a good workout—*not* sharp and agonizing pain.

Typically you'll have some muscle achiness immediately following a workout; alternatively you may experience something called **delayed muscle soreness** from twenty-four to forty-eight hours following your last exercise session. This will occur after your first few workouts, but if you break in slowly, the amount of soreness should be minimal. As time goes on and your muscles become used to working out, it should disappear altogether.

Soreness is caused by internal swelling and microscopic tears in your muscle tissue. When body builders speak about being ripped, they're not kidding! When these tiny rips repair, your muscles become stronger, firmer, and shapelier. In fact, it's this constant cycle of tearing down and building up that helps you achieve maximum tone.

However, no workout should make you feel as though you just ran your body through the garbage disposal. If you can't walk down the stairs under your own power or stand completely upright the day after a target toning session, you've most definitely overdone it! Go easy for the next few days, and do as much gentle stretching as you can. Fortunately, if you follow the isolation routines at the back of each target toning chapter and the workout procedures we've outlined for you, this shouldn't be an issue.

HIP GIRTH (INCHES)	PERCENT FAT	HEIGHT (INCHES)
32	10	72
	14	70
34	18	68
36	22	66
	26	64
38	30	62
40	34	60
	38	58
42	42	56

Human Kenetics Publishers, Inc.
Sensible Fitness, 2nd Edition
Jack Wilmove, Ph.D. CR-1986

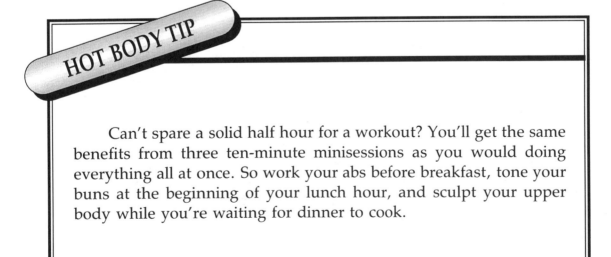

HOT BODY TIP

Can't spare a solid half hour for a workout? You'll get the same benefits from three ten-minute minisessions as you would doing everything all at once. So work your abs before breakfast, tone your buns at the beginning of your lunch hour, and sculpt your upper body while you're waiting for dinner to cook.

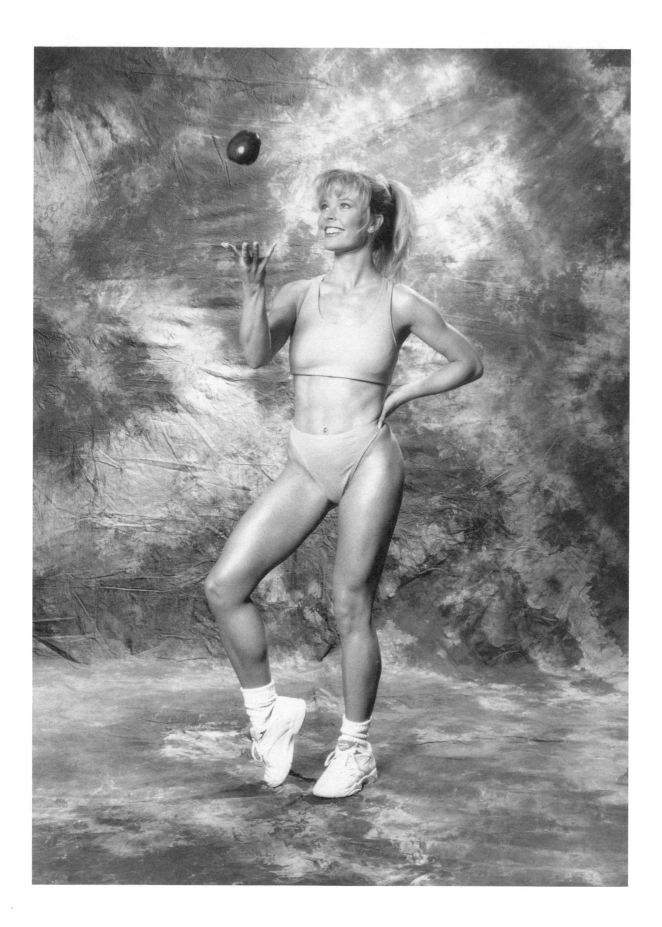

Buns of Steel Basics

Think about the dedicated jogger who looks as if she couldn't lift a heavy box if her life depended on it. Sure she can run for miles, but that doesn't mean she's the picture of fitness. That's because optimal fitness is really the sum of four parts: strength, stamina, flexibility, and nutrition. Conventional wisdom held that it was enough just to eat a low-calorie diet and strengthen your heart and lungs with cardiovascular exercise. Though that went a long way toward weight loss, it did nothing for the tone and appearance of the muscles. And many aerobically fit people couldn't touch their toes! Thank goodness we know better now. Think of total fitness as a jigsaw puzzle—if there's one piece missing, your puzzle is not complete. When you slip the missing pieces into place, you've got the complete picture of health. And one that looks darn good in the mirror, too!

Twenty years ago embarking on a weight-loss program meant stringent dieting. Ten years ago it meant a couple of hours a week on a treadmill, stair climber, or some other form of cardiovascular training. Now, however, recent research has confirmed the real secret to *long-term* weight loss. And it may surprise you.

The secret? Strength training in general and target toning in particular. Ironically, women have always shied away from *any* type of strength training because we were afraid it would make us bigger. Now it seems we've stayed away from the very thing that will help us lose weight *and* reshape our bodies. Not only does the process of strength training burn up a large amount of fat and calories, it adds sexy, healthy muscle so your metabolism doesn't slow down the way it does as defense against starvation when you attempt to drop weight through dieting alone.

Consider this research study done at the University of Massachusetts: Researchers compared weight loss and body changes in sixty-five subjects, some of whom dieted, some of whom dieted and did aerobic exercise, some of whom dieted and strength trained, and some of whom dieted in combination with strength training and aerobic exercise. The result? The largest weight loss was reported by the group who dieted and strength trained. In fact, the average weight loss in that group was nine pounds, 109 percent from fat. How is it possible to lose more than 100 percent of fat? By gaining muscle through exercise as you selectively reduce fat.

Of course, we're not suggesting you abandon your aerobic workouts. On the contrary, aerobic exercise builds stamina, reduces stress, and ultimately contributes toward lasting weight reduction. What we *are* saying is this: Aerobic exercise (and a low-fat diet) is not the be-all and end-all when it comes to lowering body fat. Any sensible, safe, and effective weight-loss program must also include target toning.

Why is target toning so effective as a fat-loss tool? It's high-intensity training that brings about the biggest gains in muscle and the largest losses in fat. Unlike many other "strength" training systems that call for a high number of repetitions and light resistance, target toning involves doing eight to fifteen repetitions with a resistance (dumbbell, ankle weight, exercise band, or your own body weight) heavy enough to stimulate significant muscle growth. This muscle gain is an important contributor to ongoing fat loss: for each pound of muscle you pack onto your frame, you speed up your resting metabolism by 50 calories, so you burn more calories even when you're not exercising. *You heard us right.* Add one pound of muscle and you'll burn an extra 350 calories a week without *any additional effort.* This makes it easier to drop unwanted pounds in the future and keep off excess weight permanently.

However, since your goal is to reshape your body, your workouts must go beyond weight loss. Just becoming thin doesn't necessarily mean you'll look good in a bathing suit or a tight dress. You want firm buns, sleek thighs, and a flat stomach; you want a lower body you can be proud of and an upper body to match! Well, target toning can do that for you, too. Target toning can actually change the shape of your body. It allows you to isolate one muscle group at a time and work it with a series of carefully designed, amazingly effective exercises. Think of the control that gives you! You can actually remodel any area you choose, turning trouble zones into prime assets.

The best part is, you don't have to let exercise take over your life in order to create your perfect body. If you target tone a muscle for ten minutes, three times a week, you will begin to see positive changes in about four weeks. Most people can totally remodel an area in about two months' time with consistent training.

If you have a particularly stubborn trouble zone, you can increase your toning sessions to fifteen or twenty minutes in duration. If you're looking for a quick, full-body tone-up, you can work every muscle in your body in just forty-five minutes a week with three fifteen-minute sessions. If you're short on time, you can get by with as little as five minutes of target toning a day and still see results. The point? You can adapt the process of target toning to fit your individual needs and life-style.

Another reason for doing target toning (as if you needed another one!) is increased strength. You'll notice—perhaps after your very first workout—how much easier it is to do everyday things such as twisting the top off a jar, moving furniture, and lifting bags of groceries. And, you'll experience other positive changes you may not readily connect with increased strength. For example, strengthening your lower back, upper back, and abdominal muscles will improve your posture. Because you'll be able to stand up straighter, you'll appear thinner, more attractive, and more confident. Another example: That weak ankle that used to wobble and ache after a day on your feet will no longer bother you because stronger calf muscles will offer more support to your ankle joint.

Now that you know all the great things regular target toning can do for you, let's dispel the biggest myth about it (and about any other type of strength/resistance training, for that matter). Once and for all: *Target toning will not make you big and bulky!* In order for your muscles to reach epic proportions, you'd have to spend hours and hours in a gym, five or six days a week, and hoist gargantuan weights. Even then there's a good chance you wouldn't bulk up! Very few women possess high enough amounts of testosterone (the male hormone responsible for increasing muscle size) to add much girth to their arms, legs, or any other muscle.

In fact, this is what will happen if you're consistent about target toning: You'll go down a few dress sizes. Target toning will whittle away at your proportions because your muscles will become tighter, more compact, shapelier, and more attractive. Your clothes will be looser even though your weight may not change much. Why? Muscle is denser than fat, which means it takes up less room. (One pound of muscle will take up a third less space than a pound of fat.) In effect, you will redistribute your weight so your physique will take on more perfect proportions. If, on the other hand, you're too thin, adding new muscle will build sexy new curves.

Putting Aerobics in Perspective

Over the past thirty years there has been a rallying cry around aerobics, to the point where, in some circles, the words *fitness* and *exercise* have become synonymous with *aerobics*. And it is true, aerobic exercise *can* do a lot for your health and appearance. Cardiovascular exercise, performed on a regular basis, will improve your stamina for fitness, sports, and daily activities. It can help lower your blood pressure and cholesterol level. It's an invaluable tool for helping individuals recover from heart disease. In order to achieve a reasonably good level of fitness, you need to do at least a minimum of three twenty-minute sessions a week. By doing this minimum you can improve your stamina, decrease your blood pressure, and ease your stress level.

What all the aerobic exercise in the world *won't* do is help you shape your body into the form you've always wanted. For that you need target toning. Aerobic exercise will, however, enhance your target toning efforts in several ways. If you use your aerobic workout as a pretarget toning warm-up, it will send oxygen-rich blood flowing into all your muscles. Your muscles will be warmer, so they'll be more pliable and less likely to get pulled or strained in the course of a target toning. You'll also find that as a result of doing your cardiovascular exercise before you target tone, your recovery time between sets will be much faster, and the sets themselves will be more effective. (If you prefer, it's not wrong to do your aerobic training after target toning but we do feel there are distinct advantages to doing things in the order we recommend in chapter 3.)

Aside from making your workout better, the aerobic portion of your workout will in itself make you look better. It will help you burn calories and lift the layer of fat covering your newly formed muscles. A combination of target toning, aerobic exercise, and a reduction in fat intake will yield quicker results than target toning alone.

Finally, a consistent program of cardiovascular exercise will just plain make you feel better. There's plenty of evidence to show that aerobic activity increases mental activity, and you'll find that for several hours following your aerobic session you will be much more clearheaded, your thought processes more acute. On the physical side, it will improve your capacity to deal with the rigors of everyday life, and you'll find yourself experiencing fewer down periods during the day. Workoutwise it will leave you feeling more energetic on the days you might otherwise have felt too sluggish to exercise.

When it comes to choosing an aerobic activity, let imagination and variation be your guide. Go for a brisk walk on a warm day, funk-aerobics class on a cool day, or a competitive game of racquetball any day! You can ride a stationary bike in front of the TV at home, walk to work, find a group of friends to run with, or pop in a step video at home. Anything that gets your heart rate pumping and makes you breathe hard for a period of twenty minutes or more qualifies. The possibilities are endless.

The chart on page 20 gives you a range of calories you'll burn during various activities. If you do the activity at a lower intensity you'll be toward the lower end of the calorie burning range, and if you work at a higher intensity you'll be toward the higher end of the calorie burning range. A good way to gauge this is by where your exercise pulse falls in your target heart rate zone. The number of calories you burn during physical activity depends on how much you weigh, so if you're lighter than 130 pounds you'll burn fewer calories than indicated on the chart, and if you're heavier than 130 pounds your calorie burn will increase.

CALORIE BURN CHART FOR AEROBIC ACTIVITIES

ACTIVITY	CALORIES BURNED* IN 30 MINUTES
Box Aerobics	130–180
Cross-Country Skiing	175–360
Cycling	130–210
Dance Exercise (Aerobics)	175–270
Jogging (10–12-minute miles)	255–300
Jump Rope	265–340
Rowing	130–230
Running (faster than 10-minute miles)	330–400
Sliding (lateral movement training)	302–380
Stair Climbing	243–288
Step Aerobics	184–225
Swimming	130–230
Walking	130–170

*Based on 130-pound body weight.

Stretch Your Limits

Flexibility refers to how tight or loose you are—in other words, the range of motion through which you can move your joints and muscles. Your level of flexibility depends upon several things: your age, your activity level, the structure of your joints. But even if you haven't touched your toes in years, you can improve your flexibility through stretching. Will taking those few extra minutes to work on your flexibility contribute to your success in your campaign to reshape your body? You bet it will! Its contribution may not be readily apparent, however, so we'll explain:

Most experts now believe that tight muscles are more likely to tear or pull. Consequently poor flexibility is thought to be one of the major causes of sports and fitness injuries. And if a muscle is injured that means it can't be used in target toning exercises. It will take you that much longer to create the body of your dreams if you're constantly waiting for a pulled muscle to heal.

Besides, limbering up the back of your thighs and your lower back will often help you reduce or avoid lower back pain. You'll stand up taller and your body alignment will become more natural. Being free of this discomfort that plagues most adult Americans will enable you to do more of the things you enjoy. This holds true with any muscle group you make looser. Wouldn't you love to be free of "phone neck" or "computer fingers"?

Stretching also seems to relieve delayed muscle soreness, the extreme ache that often occurs twenty-four to forty-eight hours after a tough workout. Many experts believe that stretching eases the pressure in the joints and muscles caused by a buildup of fluids surrounding the damaged area and thus speeds up recovery. It isn't known exactly how this works, but suffice to say the world's top athletes and dancers all stretch to remedy their aches and pains.

We like to stretch after each workout because it makes us unwind and ease back into reality. After a hard workout—or a hard day—what could be better than a quiet, relaxing stretch?

Eating to Excel

How many times have you stood in front of a mirror and said, "I start my new diet right now"? Well, as you've probably already learned for yourself, dieting can never and will never be the cure-all for your figure problems. Once and for all: *Diets don't work.* Ninety-five percent of people who lose weight through diet alone gain back all the weight they lost within a year. Even worse, it's harder to lose weight the next time around because you've lost valuable muscle tissue and slowed down your metabolism. But let's say you're one of the lucky 5 percent that manages to keep off the weight. If you've done so by dieting alone, what you end up with is a slightly smaller version of the body that started you dieting in the first place; you've done nothing to tone and define it.

Forget dieting! To get the most out of your fitness program, you want to practice good eating habits rather than count calories. Proper nutrition will give you more energy for your workouts and provide the building blocks to construct your ideal body. Here are some basic nutritional guidelines that will help you transform your body into toned, sleek, and healthy—not just slim.

• *Get most of your calories from complex carbohydrates.* Your body and brain derive most of their energy from carbohydrates. (Those of you who have tried high-protein, low-carbohydrate diets know how sluggish these can leave you feeling.) Carbohydrates come in two forms: simple and complex. Simple carbs are found in refined and natural sugars and are simple to break down, so they yield immediate energy. Complex carbohydrates, such as those found in grains and vegetables, release energy into your system more gradually.

Try to stay away from the simple sugars found in cookies, cakes, and candy. These give you a quick burst of energy but stimulate the release of large amounts of insulin, which sends you crashing back down, craving more energy and more food. You end up eating more and consuming lots of extra calories. If you feel you need some quick energy, have some fruit. The fiber content of fruit fills you up while the sugars give you energy. Few fruits contain more than one hundred calories. Just stay away from avocados and coconuts. They're high in fat.

As for complex carbs, all vegetables are fair game. Pastas, whole-grain breads, and potatoes are particularly appealing, as they all provide you with nonmeat sources of protein. One potato can supply 10 percent of your daily protein requirement and a serving of pasta, up to 15 percent.

• *Limit your fat intake.* You can follow all the exercise advice in this book and still not reach your full potential if you have a layer of fat covering your beautifully carved muscles. Ridding yourself of excess body fat will unveil your sculpted shape. Pay attention to food labeling, and try to stay away from foods that get more than 30 percent of their calories in the form of fat. Reducing your fat intake to this level doesn't have to be a drastic affair. Little changes go a long way. Forgo that extra pat of butter on your dinner roll, sauté vegetables in chicken broth instead of oil, and order dressing, gravies, and sauces on the side so you control the portion sizes.

• *Protein builds muscle.* You need a certain amount of protein in your diet in order to build your new, more shapely physique. Stick with fish and lean meats such as white turkey or chicken. Avoid the skin of the chicken or turkey, and stay away from fried foods, which soak up fat. And remember, protein doesn't come only from animal sources. Whole grains, beans, and some other vegetable sources—for example, potatoes and soy—also supply significant amounts of protein without adding a ton of fat to your diet.

But no matter what you put in your mouth, the best way to maintain big changes in the shape of your body is through a combination of target toning, aerobic exercise, and stretching. Here's something else to chew on: Exercise in general leads to a sense of well-being that translates into a sense of control. Seeing real, positive changes in your body is bound to inspire you. You'll be more aware of what you put in your mouth, and odds are you'll be less inclined to eat something you know you'll have to work off later. That's why the Buns of Steel Total-Body Workout and a proper diet go hand in hand!

HOT BODY TIP

If your schedule is so packed you find it hard to squeeze in a workout, try this: Schedule an appointment to exercise just as you would any other important obligation. For instance, write down on your daily calendar, "Wednesday, 3:30 P.M.: Power walk for 20 minutes. 10 minutes target toning exercises." Pencil in at least three thirty-minute sessions each week.

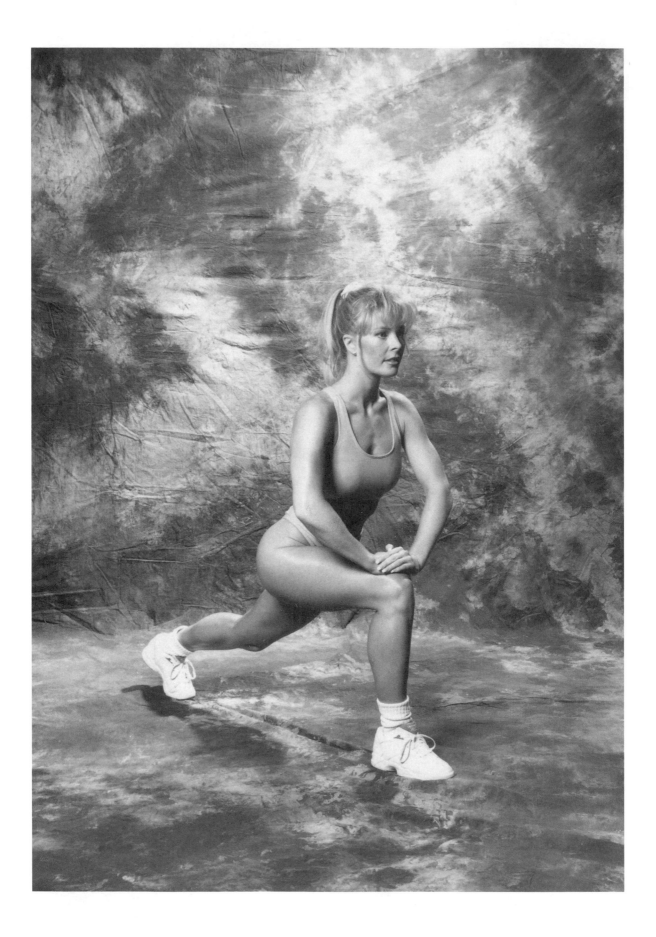

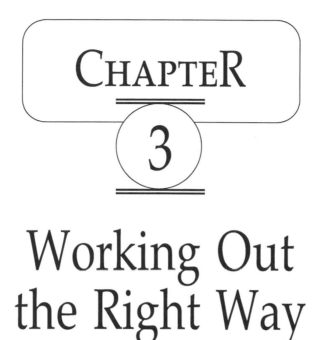

CHAPTER 3

Working Out the Right Way

A properly designed workout shouldn't leave you feeling completely exhausted. On the contrary, you should feel energized and ready to tackle anything. A sensible workout schedule will develop tone, strength, and stamina, yet leave you flexible and injury free. It's balanced. It's focused. And it gets results fast.

Your workout should include four essential elements: a warm-up, an aerobic activity, a target toning session, and a cooldown. Each of these is vital, and no workout program is complete if you neglect one. Get into the habit of doing a well-balanced workout, and you'll have a shapelier body without sacrificing your joints and muscles to injury or overtraining.

We're not suggesting you have to do an aerobic workout or a target toning session every time out. Since you only need to target tone three or four days a week to tighten and reshape your body, there may be days where you'll go for a walk but skip your buns, thighs, and abs routine. That's perfectly okay. On the other hand, there may be days when you decide to focus on sculpting your body and forgo any aerobics. That's okay, too.

However, you shouldn't totally ignore one for the other, and you should *always* include a warm-up and cooldown.

Ready, Set, Warm Up!

Adding a proper warm-up before an aerobic or target toning session serves the same purpose as warming up your car. Just as your car runs better if you take a few moments to allow the gasoline to flow through the engine, warming up your body increases the blood flow to your muscles, raises your body temperature, and gets your heart pumping. In other words, it prepares your body for the work at hand.

Take our advice. Begin each and every workout with a five- to ten-minute warm-up. Skipping this prep time is like *asking* for an injury. You don't have to get complicated; any activity that gets your heart rate up and, literally, makes your body warmer is an acceptable warm-up. Biking, fast walking, stair climbing, stepping, jogging, skipping rope—all of these will rev up your motor.

Marching in place is one of our personal warm-up favorites because it's so convenient. It requires no equipment, you need only a little bit of room to move around, and you can do it anywhere. All you have to do is lift up your knees and pump your arms. If you want to get more elaborate, put on some music and march to a beat. Tap your toes out to the side and then back to the center. Swing your arms from side to side across your body, press up to the ceiling, punch out in front of you—do anything as long as it's safe and gets you moving!

Move into Aerobics

There are several schools of thought on whether you should do your aerobic work before or after your target toning exercises. We like to do our aerobics first to build up a good sweat and burn some calories. Our muscles seem to move through the isolation routines more easily after a brisk walk or

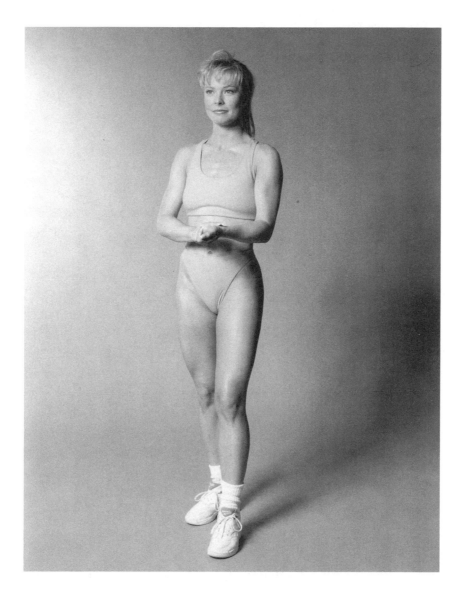

some other cardiovascular activity. However, it's not wrong to do things the other way around if that's your preference, as long as you warm up.

While the activities you do are the same, the aerobic portion differs from the warm-up primarily in terms of intensity. You warm up to ease yourself into your workout; you aerobicize to burn fat and calories, get your heart and lungs into shape, and build endurance. That's not to say you have to kill yourself in order to get results. But you do need to get your heart pumping and your muscles working in your **Training Zone** for at least twenty minutes to reap real aerobic benefits.

Your Training Zone is the minimum and the maximum workout intensity for safe and effective exercise. In other words, it's the point where you're working hard enough but not too hard. Fortunately you don't have to guess at your proper Training Zone; below we explain three ways you can gauge it accurately. Give each method a try and decide which option works best for you. The important thing is consistently to keep tabs on your aerobic work level if optimal results—particularly calorie and fat burning—are your goals.

Because your heart rate increases proportionally with the demand placed on your body, it's a good indicator of how hard you're working. The heart-rate level recommended by cardiologists, researchers, and fitness experts alike is known as your **Target Heart-Rate Range**.

Your Target Heart-Rate Range is based upon your age and fitness level. To determine where your heart rate should be during a workout, subtract your age from 220 and then multiply this number by 60 and 85 percent (.6 and .85). Alternatively, you can find your age on the Target Heart-Rate Chart on the next page and check out the corresponding range. During the aerobic portion of your workout, your heart rate should fall between these two numbers. Beginning exercisers should strive to stay at the lower end, while more advanced exercisers can push themselves to heart rates near the middle to high end of their range.

To take your heart rate or pulse, use your first two fingers, *never your thumb*. Press your fingertips lightly on the top of your opposite wrist directly below your thumb, where you should feel the pulsing rhythm of your **radial artery**. Count the number of beats you feel in fifteen seconds and either multiply this number by four or check out the Heart-Rate Finder below. *This is your heart rate.*

Monitor your heart rate periodically during your workout and immediately after finishing your aerobics. If it's too high, back off a little. But if you find it's too low, get into gear!

The following chart tells you where your exercising heart rate is. To use the chart, take a 15-second pulse at your wrist or neck and find the corresponding heart rate in the adjoining column.

TARGET HEART-RATE CHART

15-SEC. PULSE	HEART RATE	15-SEC. PULSE	HEART RATE
20	80	34	136
21	84	35	140
22	88	36	144
23	92	37	148
24	96	38	152
25	100	39	156
26	104	40	160
27	108	41	164
28	112	42	168
29	116	43	172
30	120	44	176
31	124	45	180
32	128	46	184
33	132	47	188

Another way to gauge exercise intensity is to go by how you feel. The simple way to do that is known as **Rated Perceived Exertion** (RPE for short). This is a measurable way to compare how hard you *think* you're working against how hard you *actually are* working. Let us explain:

Think about doing something that's not very taxing physically, for instance, sitting here reading through this chapter or lying in bed watching TV. On a scale of one to ten, these activities are considered a one in terms of sheer physical effort. Now think of something that's very challenging to your body, such as running up a long, steep hill at an all-out pace—something you absolutely can't continue for very long. That rates a ten on the effort scale. Your training zone is somewhere in the middle of your hardest and easiest efforts, or a five to eight on the RPE scale. In other words, moderate to heavy.

As you're working out, keep the RPE scale handy and try to put a value on the difficulty of your workout. If you feel your working intensity is below a five, pick up the pace; if you feel your working intensity is over an eight, back off. After a while you won't need the chart in front of you to tune in to how you're feeling. You can simply picture it in your mind.

Rated Perceived Exertion (RPE) is a subjective scale to determine how hard you're working. In exercise testing, RPE has been found to correlate closely with heart rate and other physiological functions. Find your work level by glancing at the descriptive column in the middle and comparing your effort level to the sample activities in the far right column.

RATED PERCEIVED EXERTION

NUMERICAL RATING	SUBJECTIVE RATING	COMPARISON ACTIVITIES
0	Nothing at all	Sitting still, Reading, Listening to music, Lying down
0.5	Very, very weak	
1	Very weak	
2	Weak	Standing in line, Hailing a cab, Leisurely stroll
3	Moderate	
4	Somewhat strong	Moderately paced walk, Gardening, Calisthenics
5	Strong	
6		
7	Very strong	Brisk jog, Biking over rolling hills, Quickly climbing stairs
8		
9		
10	Very, very strong Maximal	Sprinting hard up a steep hill All-out effort

HOT BODY TIP

To sidestep injury and muscle soreness, ease into fitness activities gradually. For instance, if you take up running, don't increase your mileage by more than 10 percent a week.

The most elementary way of all to tell if you're in the proper training zone is the **talk test**. The talk test is based on how easy you find it is to carry on a conversation during your workout. It probably works best if you actually have another person to talk to, but there's no rule that says you can't talk aloud to yourself, provided you say something encouraging!

You're in the low end of your training range if your breathing is quicker than at rest but you can still carry on a normal conversation. Toward the middle of your range, your breathing will become somewhat deeper—loud enough to hear. You'll still be able to carry on a conversation, but perhaps not quite as easily. At the high end of your range, your breathing will become very deep and audible. You'll still be able to carry on snatches of conversation, although it will be somewhat difficult. If you can't speak at all and your breathing is broken and choppy, you're definitely overdoing it!

Getting into Target Toning

Target toning is the meat of your workout, the part that brings about real changes in the shape and tone of your body. After doing your warm-up and aerobics, your body is primed and ready to go. It's time to zero in on those trouble zones! Before you begin your target toning routine, spend a few minutes planning. What are your goals for today? What equipment do you need? There's nothing worse than breaking the rhythm of your session because you have to stop and learn how to do an exercise from scratch or hunt around for your five-pound weights.

Take some time to read through the individual exercise descriptions and the isolation routines. Decide what parts of your body you want to target, the routines you'll be doing, and gather together all the equipment (if any) you'll need *before* you start. You can do this advance work the night before a session if you want or whenever you have a little spare time. Taking these few extra minutes to prepare properly will really make a difference in your workout.

We recommend that when first starting out, you stick to the ten-minute isolation routines located in the back of each target toning chapter. These are designed to zero in on a particular area of your body and shape it to perfection. Do the exercises in each routine in the order listed, and perform each one exactly the way it's described. After you've been working out for a few weeks, you can branch out into the fifteen- and twenty-minute routines and then, if you wish, begin using the specialty routines you'll find in the "Putting It All Together" chapter. Once you feel comfortable with the correct form of the exercises and have an instinctive idea of how they should feel, you can make up routines geared specifically to your goals.

How hard should you work during target toning? Just as you did with your aerobics, you should strive to get into your proper Training Zone. This is something you can measure by the amount and difficulty of repetitions you perform each set. Your aim in target toning is to do eight to fifteen repetitions of each exercise with good form. You're at the high end of your training range if you really have to push it to get to eight reps yet you can still do the exercise properly. If you can't keep proper form, ease up until you can. At the low, or less intense, end of your range, you can make it through fifteen reps yet still feel challenged. Remember, the key here is not only the number of repetitions you perform, but also the *quality of effort*. You must feel your muscles contract strongly in order to stimulate a change in them, so don't be afraid if a weight feels a little heavy or a particular exercise variation really makes you work.

If you're new to target toning, it's advisable to stay at the less intense end of your training range to head off severe muscle soreness. Give your muscles a chance to learn the ropes. However, once those fifteen repetitions are no longer challenging, you've got to make the exercise more advanced by adding resistance or changing the exercise. If you're a more experienced exerciser, you can start off with a more intense workout. The point is, if you give each individual exercise your best effort, your overall workout will yield results.

One important safety note: If you do choose to do your aerobic work first, cool off for a few minutes before you begin target toning. Allow your heart rate to slow to under 120 beats per minute before moving to any floor work where your head is below your heart; you'll avoid dizziness and weakness and, in extreme cases, fainting.

That's all we're going to say about target toning for the moment. You'll find plenty more specifics in the target toning chapters and throughout the rest of this book.

Cooldown and the Final Stretch

Whew! You did it! You roared through a tough target toning session, not to mention twenty minutes or more of aerobic exercise. You're almost there, but you're not quite finished yet. Spend a few minutes to let yourself unwind after a workout session. You've earned it.

Think of the cooldown as exactly the opposite of a warm-up yet equally as important. Just as your body needs to prepare for training, it also needs to come down after a hard workout. Anyone who has ever stopped short after a workout and felt a little light-headed knows exactly what we're talking about.

Always do three to five minutes of a slow walk, easy jogging, or pedaling with light tension on your bike after a workout session. (Choose another cooldown activity if you prefer.) Physiologically speaking, this will do a lot for you. These gentle, rhythmic body movements act as a pump to get the blood flowing away from your muscles and back to your heart. This will prevent cramping, dizziness, nausea, and sudden changes in blood pressure. It may also save you from extreme muscle soreness or injury.

Your cooldown period is also a good time to mentally review your training. It's satisfying to think about how good it felt to push yourself a little and how each workout brings you one step closer to success. You may want to make plans for your next session!

As you're cooling down, take your heart rate every minute or so. (Review "Target Heart Rate-Range," page 28.) When it goes below 120 beats per minute you can stop moving. In general, the better shape you're in, the faster this will occur. (You can substitute the RPE or talk test method if you wish. Cool down until you are in your "easy" zone.) Once your heart rate has slowed sufficiently, move on to the final stretch.

You may be tempted to skip your postworkout stretch, but don't. It's a great way to make a calm transition out of your workout mode and into something else. Many experts believe that regular stretching helps you avoid injuries and perhaps even muscle soreness. Besides, you'll *look* better if you stretch consistently: loose, limber muscles allow you to stand long, strong, and tall. Just think of the graceful dancer stretching at the barre.

Stretching increases your flexibility by extending the range of motion your joints and muscles can move through. You may have heard that it's better to stretch before a workout, but we think it's more essential to stretch at the end. When your muscles are warm from exercising, they're more pliable, so you'll get a more extensive stretch. Besides, you're more likely to injure yourself when you attempt to lengthen a preworkout muscle that's tight and cold.

If you're not exactly a rubber band when you first begin stretching, take heart. Everyone can improve flexibility with regular stretching. Here's our favorite stretching routine. Follow in order and hold each stretch for twenty- to thirty-seconds.

Buns of Steel Postworkout Stretch

Low Back "Double Knee" Hold

Lie on your back and hug your knees into your chest by wrapping your arms around the back of your thighs *underneath* your knees. You may rock gently from side to side to massage out muscle kinks and increase the relaxation of the stretch.

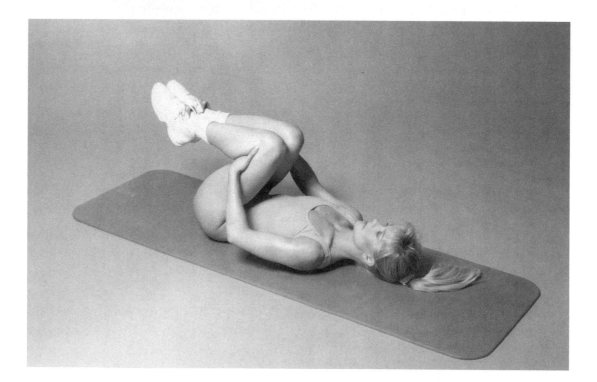

Hamstring, Calf Stretch Combo

Lie on your back with your left knee bent, foot flat on the floor. Extend your right leg, slightly bent, up over your hip and clasp your hands behind your knee. Without letting your back or buns lift off the floor, gently ease your right leg toward your chest until you feel the stretch along the back of your thigh. Flex your foot to stretch your calf. Repeat with the other leg.

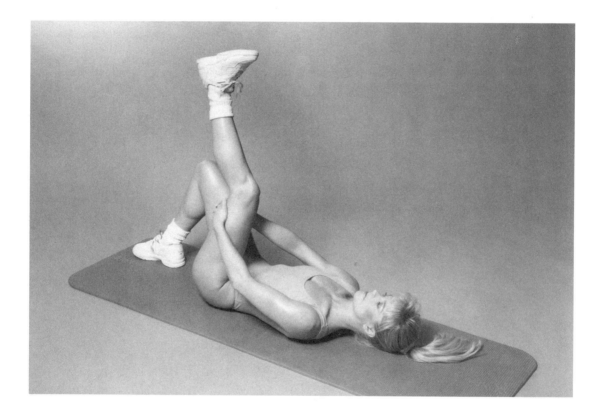

HOT BODY TIP

Americans spend over $30 billion a year on diets, yet over 95 percent of dieters regain all the weight they've lost within a year. By adding regular target toning and aerobic exercise to your efforts, you increase your chances of successful, long-term weight loss.

Hip and Lower Back Roll

Lie on your back with one knee bent and one leg straight out along the floor. Drop your bent knee across your body toward the floor. You may increase the stretch by pressing gently downward above your knee with the hand that is on the bent-leg side and extending your other arm out along the floor at shoulder level. Repeat to other side.

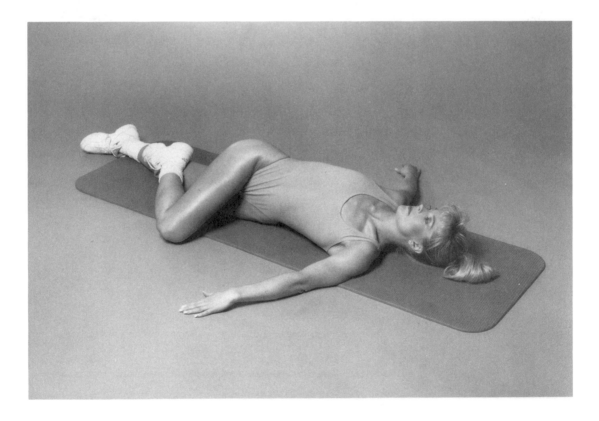

Hip and Bun "Pretzel" Stretch

Lie on your back with your right knee bent, foot flat on the floor, and your left ankle crossed over your right knee. Maintain this positioning and lift your legs off the floor. Clasp your hands around the back of your right thigh and gently pull toward you. Repeat to the other side.

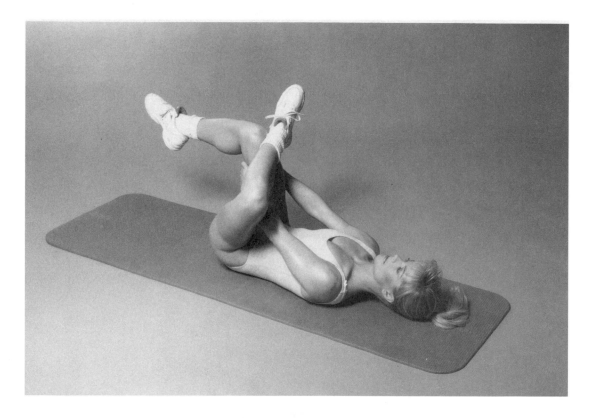

Quad Stretch

Lie on your left side with your head resting on your outstretched arm. Bend your right knee in back of you and grasp your ankle with your right hand. To increase the stretch, pull your abdominals inward and pull your tailbone forward, in line with your spine. Repeat to the other side.

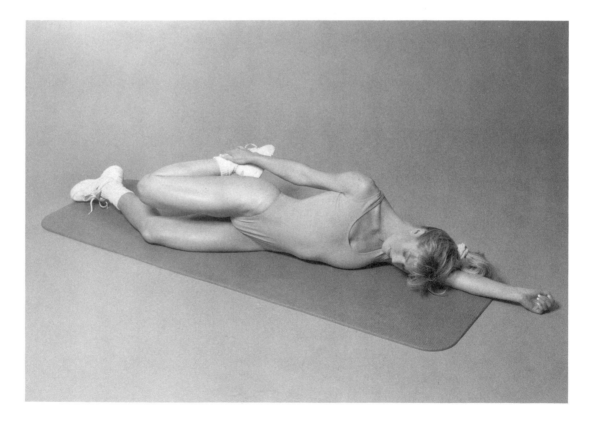

Inner Thigh Stretch

Sit up straight with the soles of your feet together and your knees comfortably dropped out to the sides. Hold both of your ankles and lean forward from your hips. Gently press your knees down toward the floor until you feel a stretch through your inner thighs. (You may also feel a stretch in your lower back.)

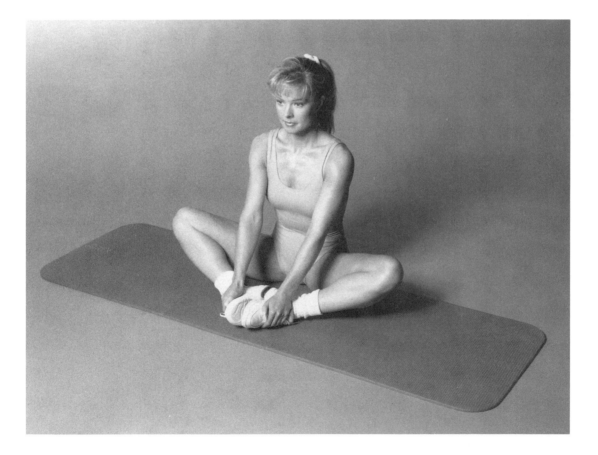

Overhead Upper Back and Shoulder Reach

Sit up straight with your legs crossed. With your palms facing away from you, lace your fingers together. Reach both arms upward and stretch tall. To increase the upper back stretch you can bend slightly to the right and then to the left.

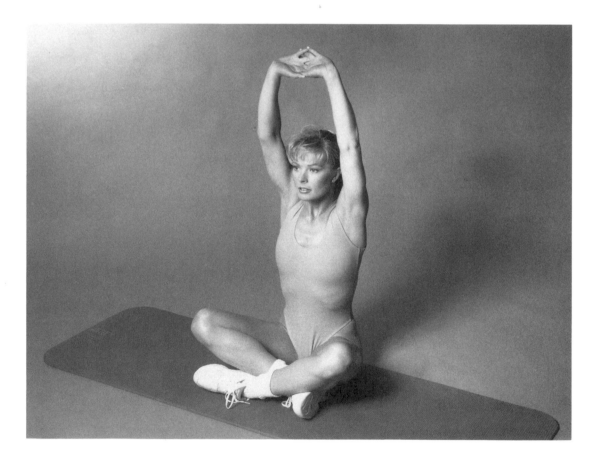

Shoulder/Triceps Stretch

Sit up straight with your legs crossed. Extend one arm across and against your body at shoulder level. Press your other palm behind your elbow until you feel a stretch in your shoulder and back of your arm. Repeat with your other arm.

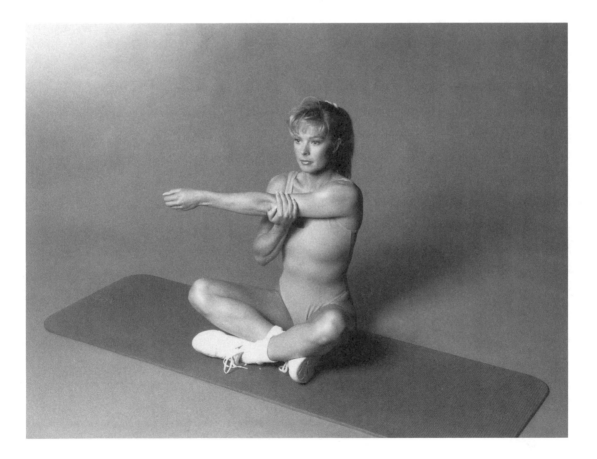

Biceps, Wrist Stretch Combo

Sit up straight with your legs crossed. Extend your left arm out in front of you at shoulder level with your palm facing the ceiling. Place your right palm on top of your left fingers and press gently downward so that your wrist bends backward and you feel a stretch through the entire length of your arm. Repeat with your right arm.

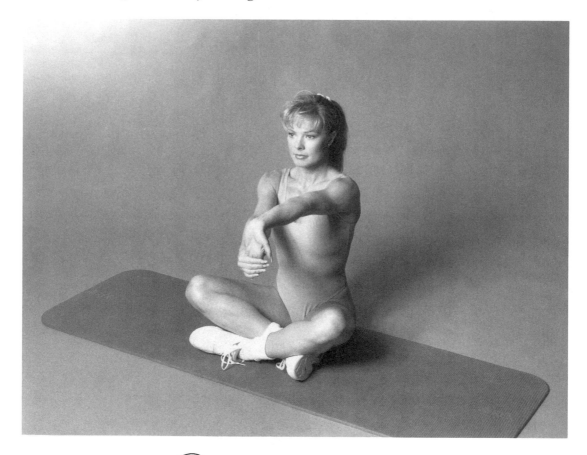

HOT BODY TIP

If you find yourself in an "aerobic rut," try something different like circuit training. And remember, cardiovascular exercise doesn't have to be a chore: a walk around an interesting museum will burn calories and stimulate your brain.

Three-Quarter Neck Roll

Sit up tall with your legs crossed. Drop your chin to your chest and gently roll through your neck by turning your head and bringing your ear toward your shoulder. Roll back to the center and then, in the same manner, roll up to the other side. Repeat two or three times.

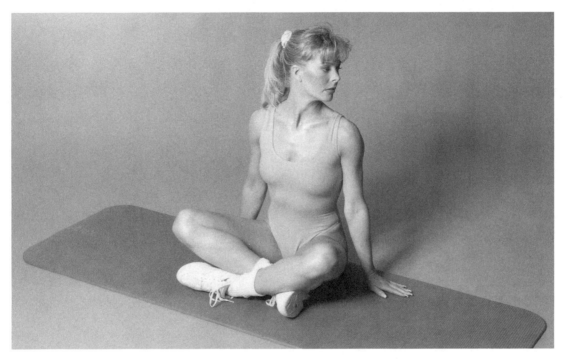

THE HOME STRETCH

• Hold each stretch about thirty seconds or until you feel a strong but gentle pull through the muscle.

• Never stretch to the point of pain.

• Don't "bounce" the muscle up and down in the stretched position. This increases your risk of injury and may actually cause the muscle to tighten.

• Make sure to breathe deeply when you stretch. You'll feel more relaxed and get more out of it.

• Try to concentrate on the muscle you're stretching while relaxing the rest of the body.

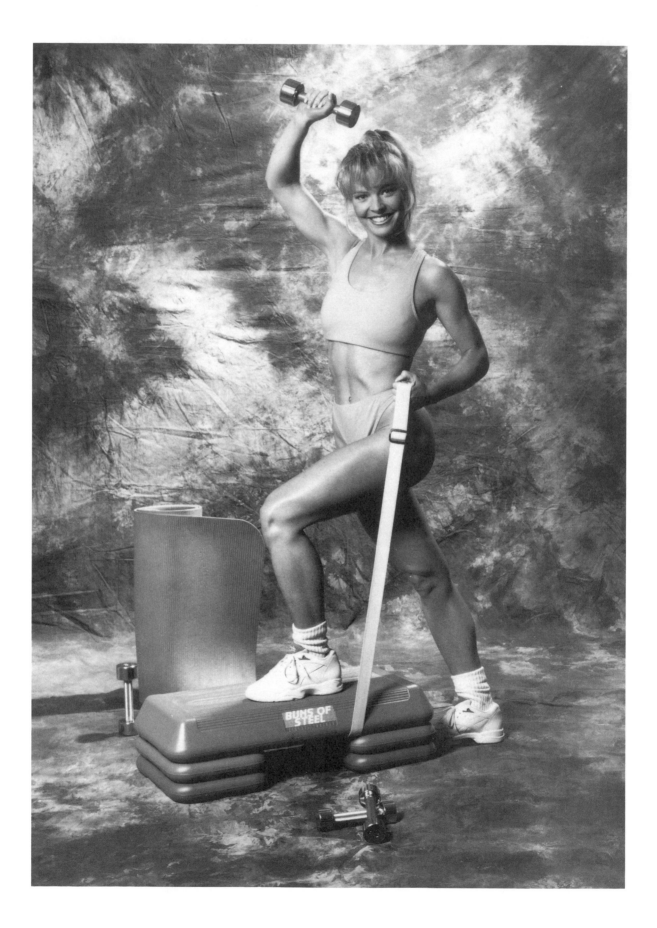

CHAPTER 4

How to Use This Book

With the Buns of Steel Total-Body Workout your target toning possibilities are endless. You can concentrate your efforts on one or two areas or give equal time to every inch of your body. That's the beauty of this program—it adapts to your needs so you can achieve the results you want in just a couple of hours a week.

The target toning chapters are arranged to isolate one group of muscles at a time. Doing routines that target a specific area of the body is a very efficient way of training, especially if you want to blast one or two trouble zones in particular. To sculpt a totally toned body, choose one routine from each chapter every time you work out.

If you're interested in doing a single routine that works the entire body or if you want to try some different types of training techniques, check out "Putting It All Together" (chapter 10). The Whole-Body, Fat Burner, and Supercircuit routines you'll find in this chapter are real time-savers and are just as results oriented as isolation workouts if you do them with the same intensity.

However you decide to use this book, we recommend you read through the information in this chapter before you jump into your target toning program. It explains the right way to go about doing your Buns of Steel Total-Body Workout and outlines the techniques and equipment you'll be using throughout. By designing a program that's appropriate for your fitness level and life-style, you'll see and feel results fast.

Each of the following target toning chapters is devoted to one area of your body, such as your buns or upper body. All of the exercise descriptions follow the same format detailed below. Take some time to read through each individual exercise description before you attempt one of the back-of-the-chapter routines.

Area Targeted: Though all of the exercises in a chapter have a primary focus on the muscle group you're targeting, they often have other benefits as well. Example: Some of the exercises in the "Buns" chapter are also great target toners for the outer thighs.

The Setup: Pay special attention to these directions. They describe exactly how your body should be positioned at the start of each exercise. The correct starting position is often the key to getting maximum results.

The Move: The photos that accompany each exercise give you a general idea of how to perform the move, but don't go by them alone. The step-by-step narration in this section contains important information to help you do the moves safely, correctly—and to maximum effect.

Mind/Body Focus: Think of these tips as a link between your body and your brain. They'll help you understand something that may be unfamiliar (an exercise) by relating it to something that's very familiar (like sitting back on a chair or rowing a boat). We also describe exactly where you should feel something when you're doing it right.

Variations: The Total-Body Workout goes beyond the basics by allowing you to adapt each exercise to suit your needs and abilities. You'll learn how to make changes when you're ready for more of a challenge or if you need to tone it down.

For Good Form and Safety: Read through this section carefully. Here's where we give you dos and don'ts to perfect your exercise form and prevent injury.

The Routines

Flip to the back of each chapter and you'll find ten-, fifteen-, and twenty-minute target toning routines that use the exercises described in that chapter. We've given you the choice of three different routines so you can arrange your Total-Body Workout around your life and *not* the other way around. Some things to take into consideration when customizing your target toning program:

• *Your present physical condition.* Although we've given you advice on how to adapt all of the routines for different fitness levels, beginners should stick to the ten-minute routines for the first couple of weeks. Once your body has gotten used to the idea of target toning, try the fifteen- or twenty-minute routines, but be sure to make the beginner's modifications we've suggested.

Consider yourself a *beginner* if you've been doing target toning or some other form of resistance training for less than three months, an *intermediate* if you've been working out for three to six months, and an *advanced* target toner if you've been working out regularly for six months or longer. Of course these are general guidelines. You may want to start with the beginner routines if you've been doing the same low-intensity workout for a long time or skip to the advanced variations if you know your body is responding to target toning very quickly.

• *Your life-style.* It seems you're always in a hurry, with a million things to do. Still, you've managed to keep up with regular workouts, so you're considered an advanced exerciser. If that's the case, you're still better off doing a ten-minute routine (with the intermediate or advanced modifications), even if you could handle twenty minutes of target toning, because you can be sure you'll fit it in. A longer routine planned might mean you'd never find the time to begin. Don't think of exercise as an all-or-nothing proposition. That ten minutes—especially if you do the exercises intensely—will get results.

• *Your emphasis.* Let's say you're pretty satisfied with your legs but want to fine-tune the look of your inner and outer thighs. Do the longer routines on the parts that need the most work and the shorter routines on the parts you're trying to maintain.

Equipment

You don't need expensive exercise equipment to do a Buns of Steel Total-Body Workout. We've designed the program around very basic exercise equipment—chances are you own most of it already. If not, you can purchase everything you need for under a hundred dollars, or you may find a suitable substitute already in your home.

• *Resistance.* Increasing the amount of tension on the muscle by adding a weight or a band is one way to up the intensity. We add resistance in our routines by using dumbbells, exercise bands, ankle weights, or simply the weight of your own body. (See "The Smart Way to Use Dumbbells," page 53, and "Exercise Band Basics," page 54.) Dumbbells and ankle weights can often be purchased for just a few dollars, and they'll last a lifetime. You'll find them in sporting goods stores and even in department or health food stores. You don't need to get fancy. Weight is weight. Soup or vegetable cans are okay to use in place of dumbbells, and they're handy because the weight is usually printed right on the label. You can also fill old detergent bottles with sand or water and weigh them on your bathroom scale. Just make sure you can get a good grip on whatever you're using, and that your wrist stays in line with the rest of your forearm when you exercise with them. If you don't have ankle weights, you can simulate their effect by applying pressure with your hands above your knee or hip joint when you're doing an exercise.

A set of exercise bands or tubes usually costs under ten dollars. If you can't find any, surgical tubing, found in many medical supply stores, is an adequate and economical alternative. However, don't be tempted to use office rubber bands. They're not strong enough to withstand much pulling and will almost certainly break if you try to exercise with them.

• *A Mat.* Anytime you kneel or lie on the ground it's a good idea to have a soft surface underneath you to cushion your joints. There are dozens of commercial exercise mats on the market, but a thick, soft towel or a folded blanket will also do just fine.

• *A Step.* Steps (or step benches, as they're sometimes called) have become quite popular in recent years. Many of the *Buns of Steel* videos use them. Most steps consist of a platform with a rubberized or otherwise no-slip surface and several sets of inserts, or "risers," that can be attached underneath the main platform to increase the step height. If you don't want to buy a step, you can use the bottom stair of a staircase for most leg exercises. Or you can prop up your head on a couple of pillows for many of the upper body exercises. You can also forgo any sort of step entirely if you wish, though in some cases the exercise will be less effective without it. (See "Step on It," page 54.)

Selecting the Right Resistance

Choosing the right resistance may take some experimentation. The resistance you use should allow you to do from eight to fifteen repetitions with good form. If it feels too light, it won't do enough to stimulate changes in your muscles, but neither should it be so heavy that you have to really struggle to lift it. When fifteen repetitions feel comfortably easy, up the resistance the smallest increment possible the next time you work out. (A workout diary is a handy way to keep track of the amount of resistance you use from session to session.)

As a general rule of thumb, beginners should start off using no external resistance and then add three- to five-pound dumbbells or one- to two-pound ankle weights when they're ready for more of a challenge; intermediates will use five- to twelve-pound dumbbells or two- to three-pound ankle weights for most exercises; and advanced exercisers will use ten- to twenty-pound dumbbells or three- to five-pound ankle weights. Of course, these are just guidelines—always go by how you feel. And keep in mind that you may use vastly different weights from exercise to exercise.

To increase the amount of resistance offered by an exercise band or tube, you can double it over once or twice, tie it off into an increasingly tighter circle, or use a thicker, less elastic band. Always use an exercise band when it's described in the basic version of an exercise.

Repetitions and Sets

A **repetition** is one complete movement of an exercise. A continuous group of repetitions is a **set**. In target toning each set consists of eight to fifteen repetitions. If you feel you can easily do more than fifteen repetitions, make the move more challenging by adding resistance or modifying it. If you struggle and break form to squeeze out eight repetitions, decrease the amount of resistance or try an easier version.

The number of sets you do depends upon the routine you're doing. Target toning works well because it uses high intensity rather than a large number of sets. Ten or so target toning sets that focus on a specific body part are done three times a week, and take about twenty minutes to complete. They are all you'll ever need to achieve the body you want.

Rest

The amount of rest you take between sets and target toning workouts is, in some ways, just as important as the amount of work you do. You need to strike a balance between just enough time so your muscles can completely recover but not so much time that you lose the focus of your workout. Usually this is from thirty to ninety seconds. When you first begin exercising you'll probably need the full ninety seconds, but as time goes on and your muscles grow stronger and firmer, you'll find you can cut this rest period down to thirty seconds or, in the case of a Fat Burner or Supercircuit routine, none at all between sets!

However, you should always rest a target area at least forty-eight hours in between workout sessions even if you're in tip-top shape. Your muscle fibers need this amount of time to fully repair following the demands target toning places upon them. That doesn't mean you can't target tone every day—simply alternate muscle groups or do a split routine as described on page 220.

Workout Intensity

There are many deceptively simple techniques you can use to change the intensity of a single exercise or an entire workout. Learning these techniques increases your options and helps you further customize your program and speed up how soon you see visible improvements.

Nearly every exercise in this book includes several variations to help you modify it for your fitness level. We've already talked about how the amount of resistance and rest you take affects intensity. Most of the other techniques fall into one of these general categories:

• *Speed of repetition.* Slowing things down is a perfect way to zero in on your buns—or any other body part—and really feel your muscles working. The slower you perform a rep, the more challenging it is. How slow is slow? Take about five seconds for both the lifting and lowering phase of the move. This is an especially potent technique for buns and abdominal exercises. On the other hand, a move done too quickly is powered by momentum rather than muscle energy. So speeding things up more than a two-second lift and a two-second lower is not a very effective way to target tone.

• *Pulses.* Many of the exercises have "pulsing" variations to increase the challenge. When you add a pulse to an outer thigh move such as side lying outward rotation (page 98), you bring your leg to the top of the movement and then lift and lower it a very small distance—no more than one or two inches in either direction—eight to twelve times. This puts continuous tension on your outer thigh muscles by forcing them to sustain a contraction.

• *Holds.* Holding an exercise at the top or the bottom of a movement often has an effect similar to a pulse, in that it increases the contraction time of a muscle and thus the effectiveness. This is known as an **isometric hold.** In other instances holding the exercise in one position for a moment increases the stretch.

• *Range of motion.* In our program you'll increase the distance you move through an exercise to make it more challenging and decrease it to make it easier. Sometimes you'll combine two or more movements together; this makes the muscle move a greater distance and thus work harder.

• *Change the angle.* Changing the angle at which you do an exercise often shifts its target toning focus. When you elevate your heels to do a squat, for instance, you place more emphasis on your legs.

• *Bilateral movements.* When you do all the repetitions with one arm or leg at a time you can concentrate your efforts on the side that's working. This increases the challenge of a move.

• *Stabilization.* Sometimes making your exercise position more stable makes things easier, and sometimes the opposite is true. When you place your feet flat on the floor to do a crossover crunch, you make it less challenging, but when you sit on a chair to perform a lateral raise, you'll definitely notice your muscles working harder!

How Long Will It Take to Do a Buns of Steel Workout?

You can do some quality toning in as little as five minutes a session (see "Split Routines," page 220). However, you'll probably see optimal results the fastest if you do at least one ten-minute routine for each targeted area three to four times a week. If you target all your muscles on the same day with one of the back-of-the chapter routines, leave yourself at least fifty minutes to complete a workout. You can trim this down by working different muscles on different days or using one of the routines from "Putting It All Together."

How Often Should You Work Out?

Most muscle groups respond best when they're worked at least three days a week. That's all the work you need to significantly reshape your body. You can do a target toning session for each area of your body all on the same day or some on one day and some the next. Just make sure each body part gets at least forty-eight hours' rest between sessions so it has time to recover.

You may have the urge to do everything at once when you first begin your Total-Body Program, but remember: More is not necessarily better. While a gung ho attitude is just what you need to mold your body into steel, you don't want to bite off more than you can chew. You'll find it much more effective to channel all that positive energy into those three or four weekly sessions!

Break in slowly. Start with the ten-minute routines and the basic exercise versions and build from there. Don't skip your warm-up in your eagerness to get into the target toning exercises. A proper warm-up (and cooldown) is important to lessen muscle soreness and prevent injury and will speed you along in your quest for a firmer, tighter, sexier body.

THE SMART WAY TO USE DUMBBELLS

• Don't attempt to lift more weight than you can handle safely.

• The proper way to pick up dumbbells: Bend your knees as you lift and hold them close to your body before you get into your starting position.

• Always keep your hand in line with your forearm so the weight doesn't place undue stress on your wrist joint.

• Whenever possible, it's a good idea to have a lifting partner "spot" all moves involving the use of dumbbells. A spotter watches you as you go through an exercise, helps you when you get tired, and gives suggestions about your technique. This is especially true when you're first learning the exercises or when increasing the amount of weight you're using.

EXERCISE BAND BASICS

• Only use bands or tubing specifically designed for exercising. (Surgical tubing is okay.)

• If your band doesn't have handles and a move calls for you to hold one end in each hand, loop the ends loosely around your palms. This prevents the circulation to your hands from being cut off.

• When a move calls for you to stand on the band with your feet hip width apart, place both feet on the center of the band and then step one foot out to the side so that there is about six inches of band between your feet. This prevents the band from sliding out from under you.

• Check frequently for holes and tears by holding your band up to a bright light. If you find any, replace the band immediately.

STEP ON IT

• Make sure risers are securely locked under the step platform.

• For lower body exercises, using the correct step height is important. Stand behind your step and place one foot on top of it. Your knee should be bent at no more than a 90-degree angle to the floor. This will be from two to eight inches, depending on how tall you are and how long your legs are. It's a good idea to use an even lower step height (where your knee is bent less than 90-degrees) or no step at all if you're first starting out.

• Be sure to wipe the sweat off your step frequently to prevent slips.

• Always place your step on a flat, nonslippery surface. Carpeted or wooden floors are ideal choices.

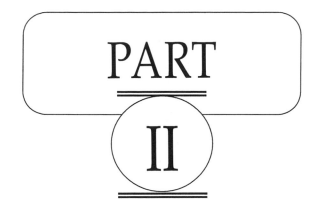

PART

II

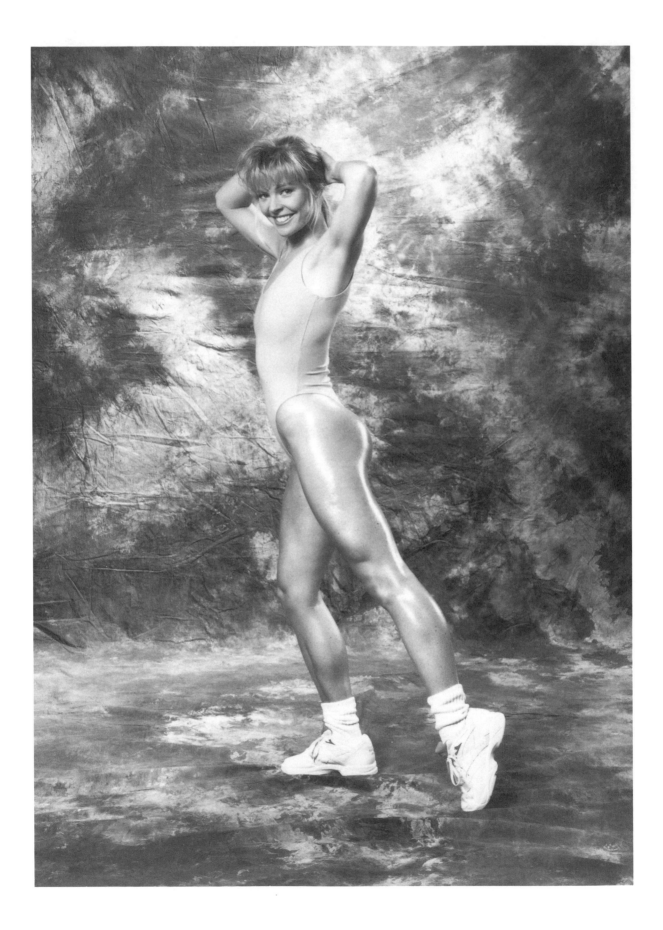

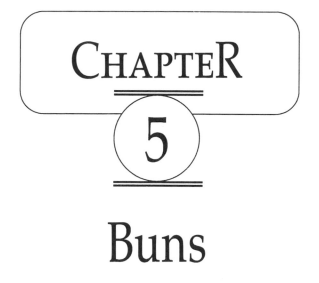

Buns

Firming and shaping buns is what put the name *Buns of Steel* on the map. For millions of women, Buns of Steel is *the* answer for sculpting a set of firm, sexy buns. Well, if you think our exercise videos are great for lifting and shaping your rear end, then you'll love the exercises in this chapter. They're guaranteed to deliver the same kind of phenomenal results.

If you want to see big changes in your buttocks, then the Buns of Steel target toning method is the way to go. Why? Because target toning your buns really works! It allows you to isolate the exact spot or spots that need changing. Even if you've tried other training methods and nothing has worked, you'll be able to chisel a better pair of buns by doing the exercises in this chapter. You *will* see and feel noticeable results with the Buns of Steel target toning method.

As you go through these moves you'll feel the muscles of your buns tightening, firming, reshaping. After a few weeks of doing these exercises consistently, you'll not only have better-looking buns, they'll also be stronger. You'll have an easier time with everyday activities like walking to the store, running to catch a bus, and climbing stairs at the office.

No matter what your body type, as long as you do the exercises in this chapter and follow the Buns of Steel program two to three times a week, you can create beautifully firm buns. Most women see significant improvements in about a month.

The major muscle in your buns is the *gluteus maximus*. Any time you stand up, climb stairs, or walk up a hill, this muscle gets a workout. So target toning your buns will not only give you a fabulous rear view, it'll also help you bound up those office stairs two at a time, and you'll never miss your bus again! When you target tone your maximus, you also work your *gluteus medius* and *gluteus minimus*. The exercises in this chapter are good for targeting these two muscles as well. You'll further isolate them with the exercises in the "Inner and Outer Thighs" chapter, so be sure to do our inner/outer thigh program, too.

This chapter provides eleven different exercises to target these muscles, then shows you how to work them into a routine that's right for *you*.

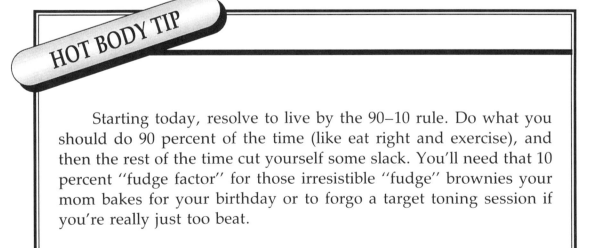

HOT BODY TIP

Starting today, resolve to live by the 90–10 rule. Do what you should do 90 percent of the time (like eat right and exercise), and then the rest of the time cut yourself some slack. You'll need that 10 percent "fudge factor" for those irresistible "fudge" brownies your mom bakes for your birthday or to forgo a target toning session if you're really just too beat.

BUNS EXERCISES

1. Squat
2. Plié
3. Squat Pulse
4. Dip
5. Basic Lunge
6. 3-D Lunge
7. Squat and Lift
8. Bun Sweeps
9. Jumpers
10. Glute Raise
11. Kneeling Glute Raise with Band

HOT BODY TIP

Even though muscle is made up primarily of protein, you don't need to eat more protein to increase your muscle tone. In fact, the average American eats twice as much protein as the body needs, and this excess dietary protein is stored as body fat. You do, however, need to eat more complex carbohydrates like bread, pasta, and whole-grain cereals to give your body the energy it needs to sail through a target toning workout.

HOT BODY TIP

Learn when to say "when." Think of your hunger on a scale of one to ten, one being so hungry you simply must eat in the next two minutes or you'll faint and ten being so full, if you eat another bite, you'll pop. Aim to wind up a five at the end of tonight's meal—and every meal—full but not too full, with a little room left over but pleasantly satisfied.

Exercise 1: SQUAT

TARGET AREAS

This is the foundation exercise for the buns and entire hip and thigh zone.

The Setup: Stand with your feet hip width apart with your hands placed on the tops of your thighs. Look straight ahead and open your chest by relaxing your shoulders backward and downward. Pull your abdominals gently in toward your spine, and maintain a natural curve in your spine.

The Move:
• Inhale and, leading with your tailbone, sit backward and downward until your thighs are parallel to the floor.
• Hold for a moment in the lowered position, exhale, and return to the starting position by pressing up through your heels.

Mind/Body Focus: Imagine you are sitting on a bench that's against a wall directly behind you. As you sit into the squat and move out of it, your tailbone should slide along the imaginary wall. You should feel the muscles in your buns and front of your thighs contract, especially as you stand up.

Variations:
• If you feel out of balance, hold on to a sturdy chair with one hand or raise your arms out in front of your chest as you squat down.
• When you're ready for more resistance, hold a dumbbell in each hand with your arms down at your sides or hands up at your shoulders.
• To place greater emphasis on your thighs, elevate your heels one to two inches on two weight plates or your step platform (with no risers underneath).

For Good Form and Safety:
• Your knees should never travel forward of your toes, so don't allow your thighs to move lower than parallel.
• Be careful not to overarch your lower back or lean too far forward.
• As you move upward, maintain good body alignment and keep your knees slightly bent, or "soft."
• If you feel this exercise in your joints (especially the knees) rather than your muscles, squat only a quarter to one-half of the way down.

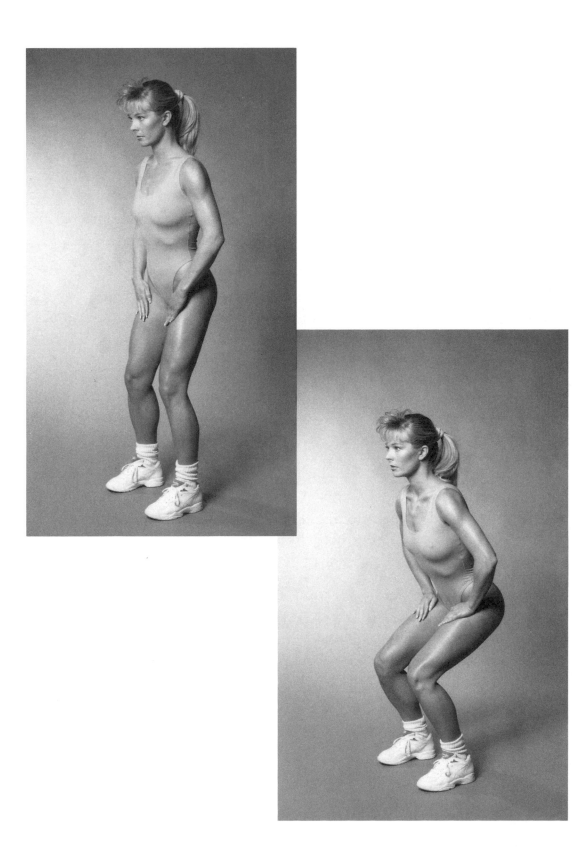

Exercise 2: PLIÉ

TARGET AREAS
Buns and entire hip and thigh area with special emphasis on the inner thigh.

The Setup: Stand with your feet a few inches wider than hip width apart, with your toes pointed out and your hands on your hips. Stand up tall and maintain your spine's natural curve.

The Move:
• Inhale. Lower your body straight downward so that your knees travel in a straight line out over your toes until your thighs are parallel to the floor.
• Hold for a moment in this down position, exhale, and return to the start.

Mind/Body Focus: Concentrate on pushing through your heels, using your buttock muscles, not your knees. You're doing this right if you feel a contraction in your buns and your inner thighs on the upward movement.

Variations:
• For more of a challenge, with both hands hold a dumbbell out in front of you at waist level.
• To add in some lower leg toning, lift your heels off the floor, lower your body, and then return your heels to the floor before standing back up to the starting position.

For Good Form and Safety:
• Don't lower so far that your knees move out in front of your toes or so you find yourself falling forward.
• Take care not to lock your knees as you reach the top of the movement.
• If you feel this move in your joints rather than your muscles, you only need to lower your thighs one-quarter to one-half of the way down.

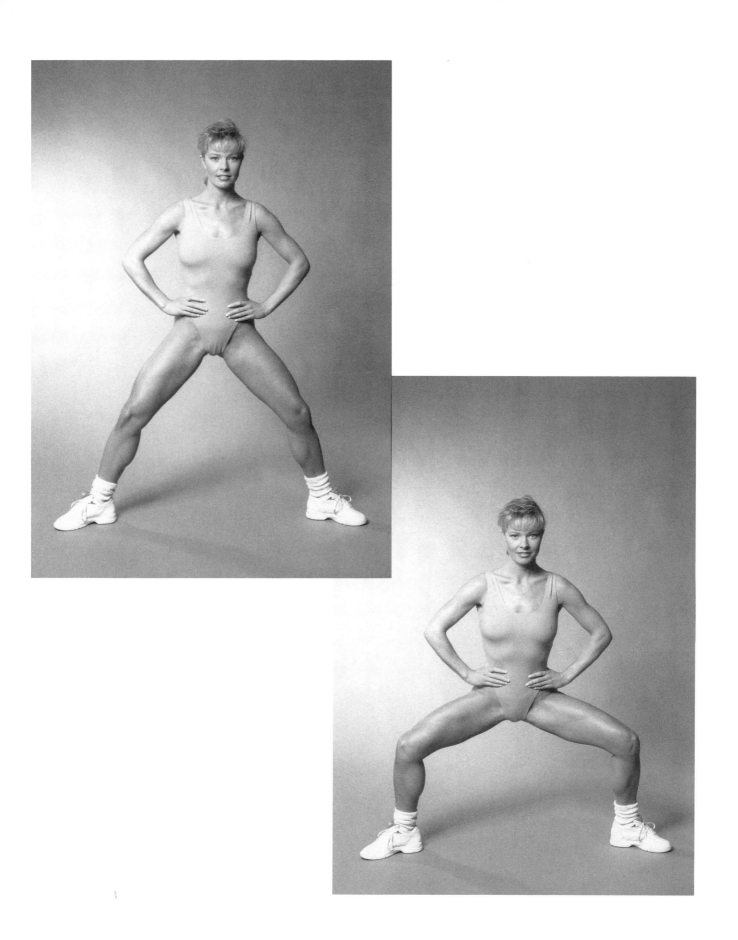

Exercise 3: SQUAT PULSE

TARGET AREAS
This exercise really blasts the buns and entire hip and thigh area.

The Setup: Stand with your feet hip width apart, and place your hands on top of your thighs. Maintain good posture and, leading with your tailbone, sit backward and downward until your thighs are parallel to the floor.

The Move:
- In this lowered position, pulse up and down a few inches eight times, squeezing your buttock muscles as you do so.
- Inhale every time you pulse down, exhale every time you pulse up.
- After the eighth pulse, move to a standing position by pressing up through your heels.

Mind/Body Focus: As you pulse, imagine you have a spring in your buttocks so that the pulsing action is smooth and continuous. When you do this exercise properly you'll feel consistent tension in your buns and front of your thighs.

Variations:
- If you feel out of balance or you want to make this exercise a little easier, raise your arms in front of your chest or hold on to a sturdy chair with one hand.
- To really challenge your inner and outer thighs, pulse in the plié position instead of the squat.
- When you're ready for more of a challenge, hold a dumbbell in each hand with your arms down at your sides or your hands up at your shoulders.
- Another way to make this more advanced: increase the number of pulse repetitions to twelve.

For Good Form and Safety:
- Be sure to keep your knees soft, especially when you stand up between repetitions!

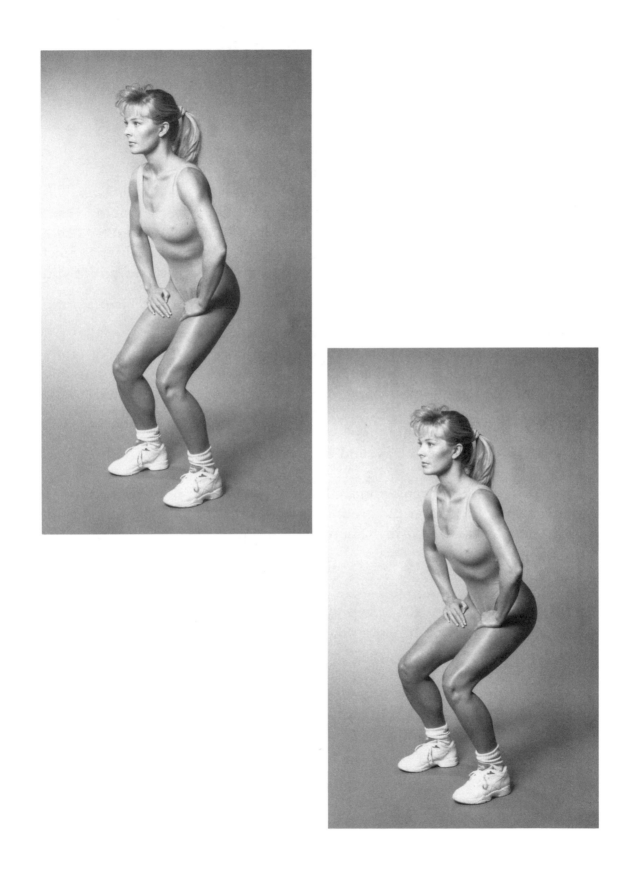

Exercise 4: DIP

TARGET AREAS
Buns, hips, and thighs.

The Setup: Stand with your feet hip width apart and, *while maintaining this hip width distance*, step your left foot back until your legs are about three feet apart in a "straddled" position. For balance, bend your front knee a little and lift your back heel off the floor. Hold your upper body in perfect alignment and, with both hands, hold on to a stable object in front of you (such as a sturdy chair) for support.

The Move:
- Inhale. Bend both knees so that your back knee almost, but not quite, touches the floor. In the finish position your back knee will be pointing straight down toward the floor and your front thigh will be parallel to the floor.
- Inhale and return to the start.
- Switch front and back legs, and do an equal number of reps.

Mind/Body Focus: Imagine you are holding two buckets of water and you're trying to place them on the ground on either side of you without spilling any. You'll feel this move in the buns and front and back of thighs, especially as you push upward.

For Good Form and Safety:
- Don't "overdip" by allowing your front knee to travel beyond your toes as you lower. If your front thigh never goes lower than parallel, you shouldn't have this problem.
- Be careful not to straighten up so much that your knees lock or bend so far forward from the hips that you feel off balance.
- Keep your upper body tall and your abs pulled in throughout. This will help secure your lower back.

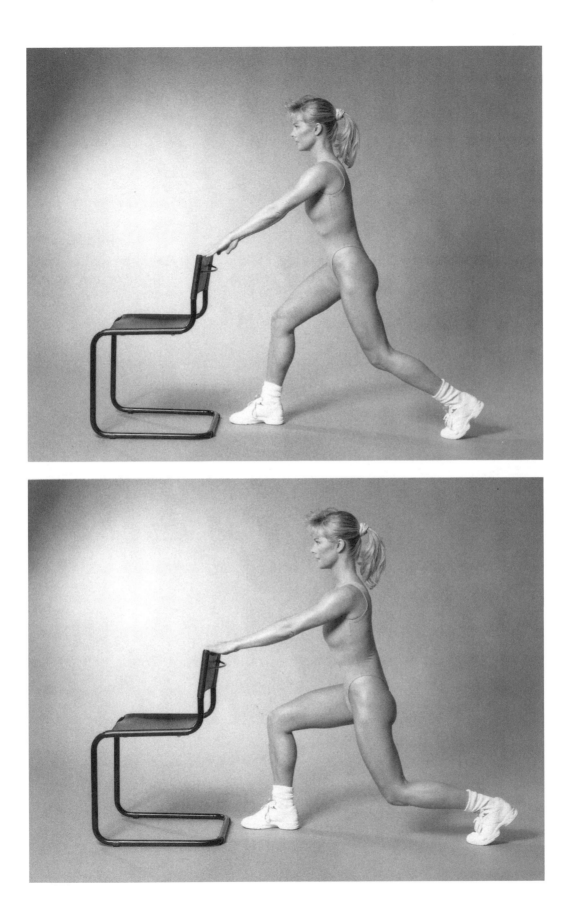

Exercise 5: BASIC LUNGE

TARGET AREAS
Buns, hips, and thighs.

The Setup: Stand with your feet hip width apart and your hands on your hips. Stand up tall by keeping your chest lifted, your shoulders square, and your abdominals tight. Maintain your spine's natural curve.

The Move: Inhale. Leading with your heel, step your right foot forward about three feet and lift your left heel.
- As your right foot lands, bend both knees so that your back thigh points straight down toward the floor and your front thigh is parallel to it. (This is exactly the same lowered position as the dip.)
- To return to the starting position, push off your right foot and "spring" back up lightly so that both your feet return to their original starting positions. Exhale as you move upward.
- Alternate working legs.

Mind/Body Focus: Pretend you are trying to step over a crack in the sidewalk. Lead with your heel so you miss the crack. You'll feel this in your buttocks and fronts of your thighs, especially as you spring upward to the starting position.

Variations:
- If you have trouble keeping your balance during this exercise, place a sturdy chair at your side and hold on to it lightly with one hand.
- To make this exercise more advanced, hold a dumbbell in each hand with your arms at your sides or place a bar across your shoulders.

For Good Form and Safety:
- *Do not overlunge*—that is, don't allow your front knee to move out past your toes.
- Avoid leaning too far forward from your hips, for this will throw your balance off.

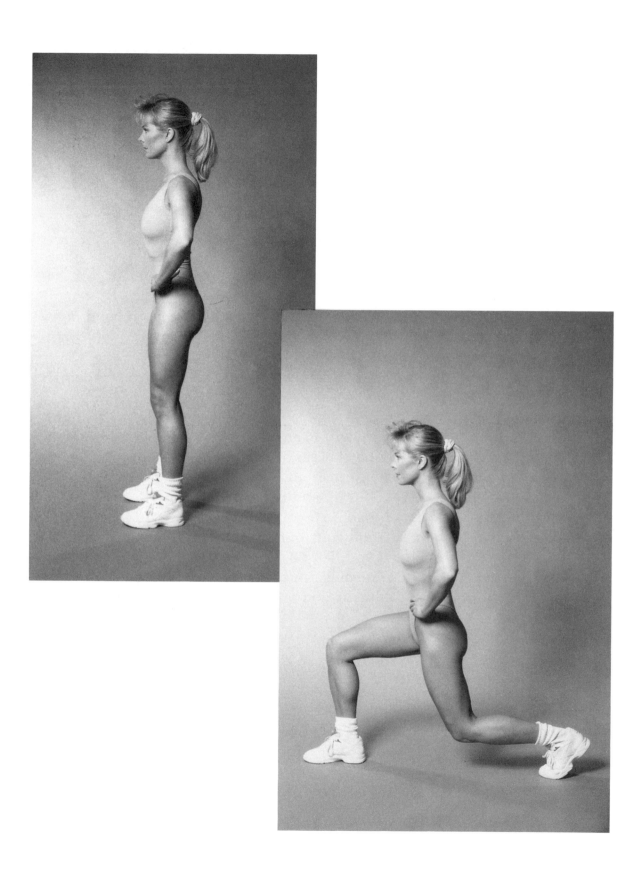

Exercise 6: 3-D LUNGE

TARGET AREAS
A complete lower body toner! Hits the buns, hips, thighs, and lower legs.

The Setup: Stand with your feet shoulder width apart. Stand up tall, with your shoulders relaxed and your chest open. Pull your abdominals gently in toward your spine.

The Move: This exercise involves a forward, side, and back lunge, all done in continuous succession. To start, move directly from the setup position into a forward lunge.

- Leading with your heel, step forward with your right leg and bend both knees so that your right thigh is parallel to the floor and your left thigh points straight down toward the floor.
- Push back up to the starting position by pressing up through your right heel.
- Move directly into a side lunge: move your right leg about six to eight inches sideways and step forward. Bend your right knee until your thigh is slightly above parallel to the floor, and keep your left leg straight. Land flat-footed with toes slightly turned out.
- Pushing off your right foot, lift up and back to the start.
- Move directly into a back lunge: step your right leg backward about three feet and bend both knees until your right thigh is now pointing straight down toward the floor and your left thigh is parallel to it. Land softly on the ball of your right foot, keeping your heel up.
- Return to the start by pushing up and forward through your left foot and straightening both legs.
- Repeat the entire sequence using your left leg as the exercise leg. Do an equal number of reps with each leg.

Mind/Body Focus: Every phase of this exercise is connected to the other phases. Done correctly there is only a brief pause as you move from one position to the next, so this exercise has a smooth, continuous rhythm. You'll feel it in every muscle of your buns, hips, thighs, and lower legs!

For Good Form and Safety:
- Every time your foot returns to the floor, make sure it lands softly so that you feel this exercise in your muscles, *not* in your joints.

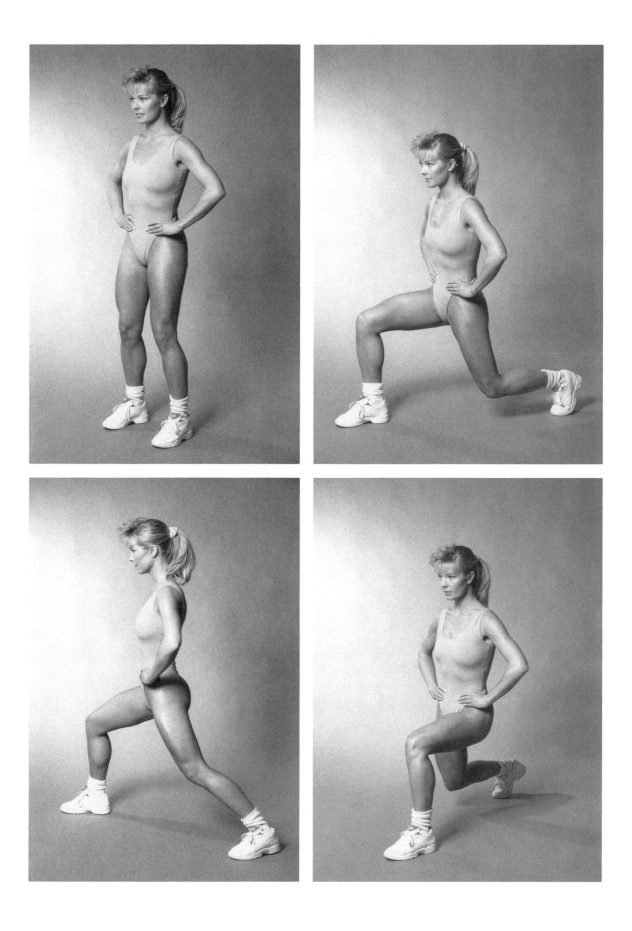

Exercise 7: SQUAT AND LIFT

TARGET AREAS
Buns, with special emphasis on the outer, inner, and front thighs.

The Setup: Stand with your feet hip width apart and your arms at your sides. Stand up tall, and keep your back aligned naturally.

The Move:
- Inhale. Step your right leg about a foot more than hip width out to the side.
- Land flat-footed and, as your right foot makes contact with the floor, bend both of your knees until your thighs are parallel with the floor.
- Exhale and push up off the ball of your right foot. Lift your right knee so that your thigh is level with your hip, and straighten your left leg.
- Step your right leg out to the side again, and repeat the move until you've completed the set.
- Switch working legs, and do an equal number of repetitions.

Mind/Body Focus: You'll feel the sideways movement in your buns and outer thighs; the upward movement in the front and inside of your working thigh.

Variations:
- When you're ready for more resistance, hold a dumbbell in each hand.
- If you find this exercise is too difficult, eliminate the lifting of your right knee and simply step back to the starting position.
- You can "power" this move by extending both arms in front of you at shoulder height as you squat down and pressing both arms back as you lift your knee.

For Good Form and Safety:
- Don't allow your nonworking knee to fully straighten or "lock."
- Good upper body posture will help you maintain your balance while doing this exercise, so remember to keep your shoulders relaxed, open your chest, and pull your abdominals in tight.
- Avoid pounding: push off and land softly and noiselessly.

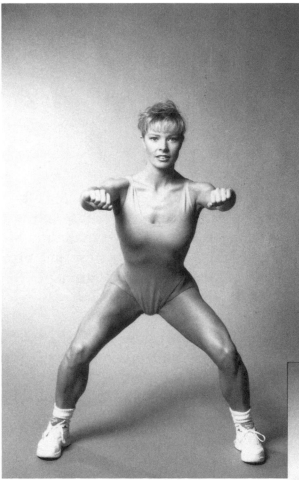

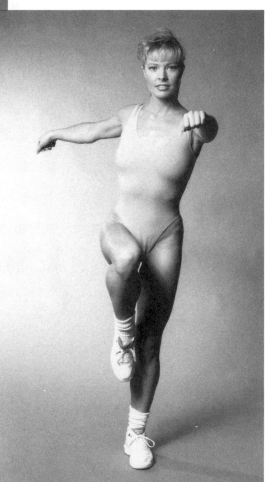

Exercise 8: BUN SWEEPS

TARGET AREAS
Buns, back of thighs.

The Setup: Stand with toes pointed slightly out and heels together. Hold your arms out in front of you at shoulder height, and rest your hands lightly on a stable object, such as a sturdy chair. This exercise will be made more effective if you stand tall, so relax your shoulders, lift your chest and rib cage, tighten your abdominals, and maintain a natural body alignment.

The Move:
- Exhale and lift your right foot off the ground, bend your knee slightly, and extend your leg backward and upward until you feel a contraction in your buttock muscles.
- Hold for a moment at the top of the movement as you consciously stand up even taller. Then inhale and return to start.
- Do an equal number of reps with your left leg.

Mind/Body Focus: Assume the posture of a tall, graceful dancer. This is a very small, precise movement. Done correctly, you'll feel continuous tension in your buttocks and down the backs of your thighs.

Variations:
- To make this move more advanced, pulse eight to twelve times a few inches up and down at the top of the movement.
- For more resistance, you may add an ankle weight or place a band around your ankles.

For Good Form and Safety:
- To avoid overarching your lower back, don't extend your leg too far back.
- Good posture is the key to making this exercise most effective. If you slouch or lean forward from the hips, your buns won't get as good a workout.

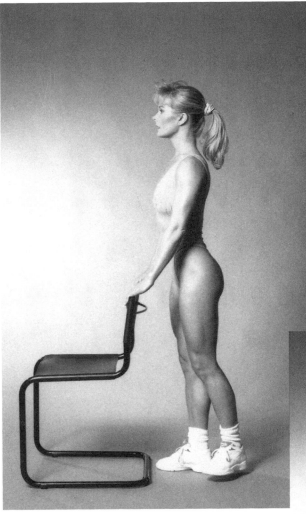

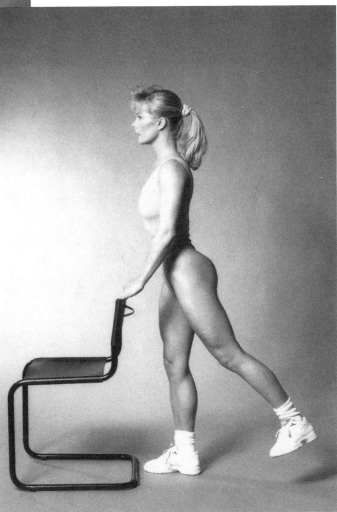

Exercise 9: JUMPERS

TARGET AREAS
Buns, hips, thighs, with special emphasis on inner and outer thighs.

The Setup: Stand on the middle of your step, facing one end with your elbows bent and your hands in fists. Maintain good posture by keeping your chest and rib cage lifted, your shoulders relaxed, and your abdominals tight.

The Move:
• Step your right leg down to the side of the step. Land heel first and roll heel to toe through the entire length of your foot until it is planted firmly on the floor. Lower your right arm to your side at the same time.
• Step your left foot down in the same fashion on the other side of the step, and lower your left arm.
• To return to the top of the step, exhale and jump up with both feet. Land softly with slightly bent knees on the top of the step. Allow your arms to swing back a little as you jump up and swing forward up into starting position as you land, so you'll touch down more softly.

Mind/Body Focus: Have you ever seen a cat jump off a high shelf and land on the floor without a sound? That's what you're striving to do with this exercise: you should touch down on the bench noiselessly and catlike. You are doing this right when you feel your outer thighs working as you step down and your inner thighs working as you jump up. You'll feel your buns working in both directions!

Variations:
• If you find this move too advanced, try it without a step. Step to each side and jump back to the middle.

For Good Form and Safety:
• Jumping a little higher than you need to helps set up a gentle landing.

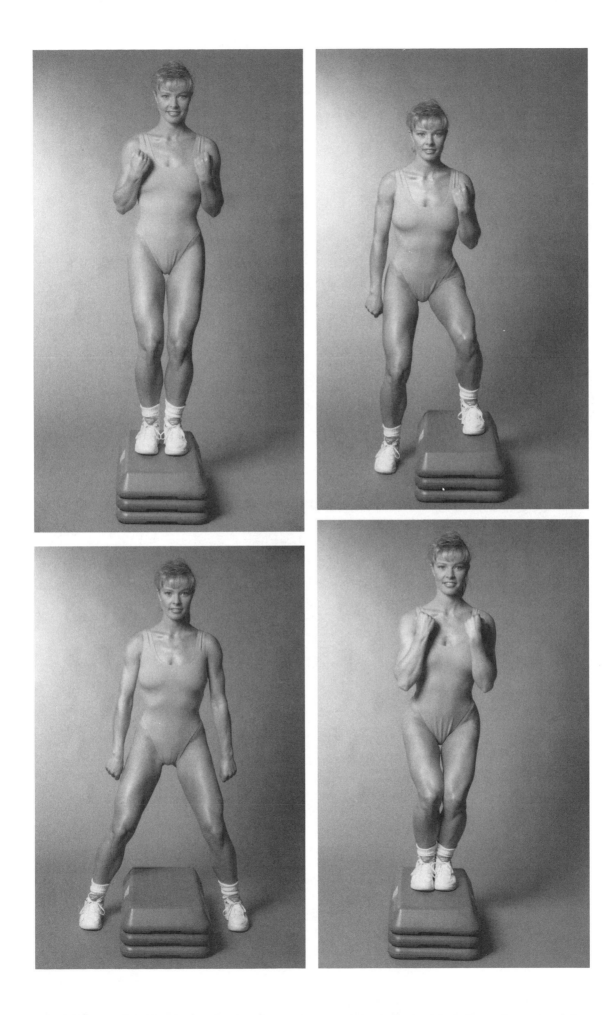

Exercise 10: GLUTE RAISE

TARGET AREAS
Target tones your buns and the backs of your thighs.

The Setup: Lie on your stomach, fold your arms, and rest your forehead on your hands. Bend your left leg 90 degrees, and press your heel flat so that the sole of your foot is facing the ceiling. To protect your lower back, go into a pelvic tilt: pull your abdominals inward, squeeze your buns together gently, and tilt your spine so that your hipbones make firm contact with the floor.

The Move:
• Exhale. Raise your right thigh one to two inches off the floor.
• Hold for a moment in the uppermost position.
• Inhale and return to the start.
• Switch legs and do the same number of reps.

Mind/Body Focus: For the setup, pull in your abs and tilt your pelvis into the floor as if you are trying to fit into a pair of jeans that are one size too small. Imagine you are squeezing a dime between your buns; try not to drop it at any point during the exercise. You'll feel a strong contraction through your buttocks and the backs of your thighs, especially if you hold at the top and squeeze your buns together.

Variations:
• For more of a challenge, pulse for a count of five in the top position.

For Good Form and Safety:
• Chances are if you feel this exercise in your lower back, you're lifting your leg too high. Keep the move small, and don't lose that pelvic tilt.

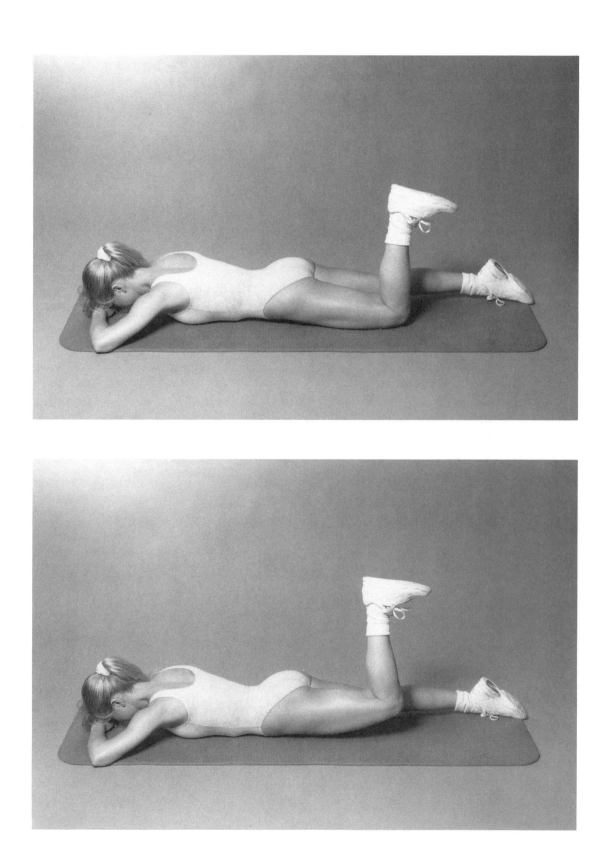

Exercise 11: KNEELING GLUTE RAISE WITH BAND

TARGET AREAS

Buns and backs of thighs.

The Setup: Tie together the two ends of about two feet of an exercise band or tube; make sure the knot is secure. Kneel on your knees and elbows with your weight distributed as evenly as possible. Align your neck with the rest of your spine by tucking your chin in slightly. Pull your abdominals in toward your spine, and allow your spine to maintain a natural curve. Place the ''band circle'' around the top of your right shoe and around the instep of your left foot.

The Move:

- Exhale. Squeeze your buns together, and lift your left leg off the floor until the back of your thigh is level with your hips. At this point the band should be taut.
- Hold for a moment at the topmost position, then inhale and lower to the start.
- Switch the band placement and do the same number of reps with your other leg.

Mind/Body Focus: Press straight up toward the ceiling. As you hold at the top of the movement, concentrate on those buns muscles—give them an extra squeeze and hold it as you lower to the start. You'll really feel this one zero in on the buns and down the backs of the thighs.

Variations:

- If you don't feel enough tension in your buns at the top of the movement, either get a stronger band or tie off a smaller circle.
- Another way to make this exercise more challenging: at the top of the movement pulse up and down one to two inches, keeping continuous tension on the band before lowering.
- To make this move easier, you can do it without the band.

For Good Form and Safety:

- Don't lift your leg any higher than hip level, and avoid arching your lower back.

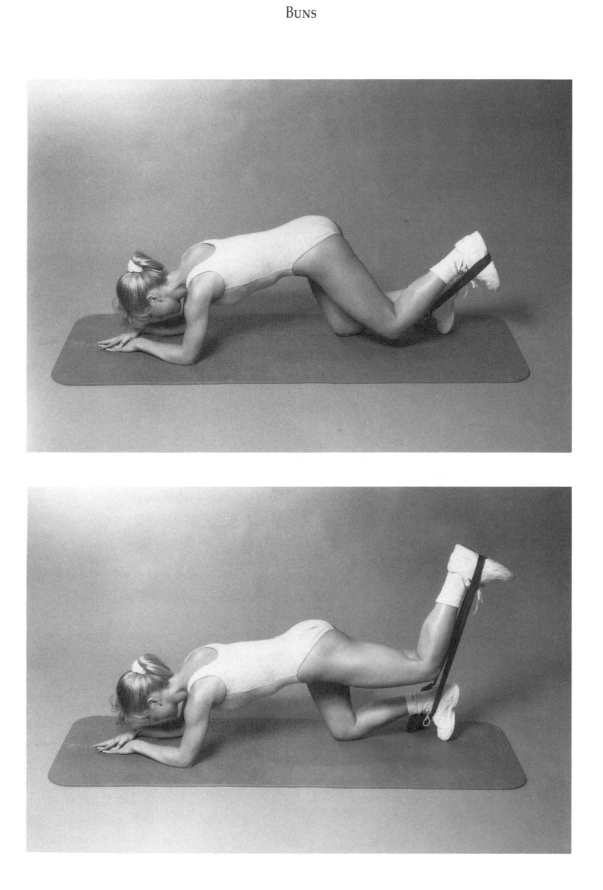

Buns Routines

Here are three buns routines you can try. Figure out how much time you want to spend target toning your buns (ten, fifteen, or twenty minutes), then adapt that routine to your level. (We've given you some suggestions on how to do that.) Once you've done our routines for a while, feel free to make up your own.

Equipment you'll need: A step, exercise band or tube, mat, and stable object such as a chair.

Optional for variations: One or two sets of risers, one or more sets of dumbbells.

How Many Reps Should I Do?

Do eight to fifteen repetitions each set. When you can do fifteen repetitions easily and with good form, move on to a more difficult variation of that exercise the next time you work out. If you find it difficult to do at least eight repetitions while maintaining good form, try an easier version of the exercise.

How Much Weight Should I Use?

When using resistance (dumbbell, ankle weight, or exercise band), choose a weight that will allow you to complete eight to fifteen repetitions with proper form. Increase the weight when you can do fifteen reps easily and with good form; if you can't get through at least eight reps, decrease the weight.

Beginners should first try each move without resistance and then add up to five-pound dumbbells and, where indicated, two-pound ankle weights, to make the moves more challenging. Intermediates, try five- to eight-pound dumbbells and two- to three-pound ankle weights. Advanced target toners add up to twelve-pound dumbbells and five-pound ankle weights. Keep in mind that these suggestions are just guidelines—always use the amount of resistance that feels challenging but allows you to complete a target toning set with good form.

How Much Should I Rest Between Sets?

Rest from thirty to ninety seconds between each exercise set. This will allow your muscles enough time to recover so they're ready to work their hardest when you do the next set, but will not be so long that you lose the intensity and focus of your workout. You'll find that as you become stronger you won't need as much rest between sets.

How Often Should I Target Tone My Buns?

For best results, target tone your buns three times a week with at least one day of rest in between each workout session.

Buns Isolation Routines

10-MINUTE ROUTINE

(BEGINNER)

ORDER	EXERCISE	RESISTANCE	SETS
1	Squat	None	2
2	Dip	None	1
3	Squat and Lift	None	1
4	Glute Raise	None	1
5	Kneeling Glute Raise	Exercise band	1

(Intermediate)

ORDER	EXERCISE	RESISTANCE	SETS
1	Squat	Dumbbells	2
2	Dip	Dumbbells	1
3	Squat and Lift	None	1
4	Glute Raise	None	1
5	Kneeling Glute Raise	Exercise band; 8–12 pulses at top	1

(Advanced)

ORDER	EXERCISE	RESISTANCE	SETS
1	Squat	Dumbbells	2
2	Dip	Dumbbells	1
3	Squat and Lift	None	1
4	Basic Lunge	None	1
5	Kneeling Glute Raise	Exercise band; 8–12 pulses at top	1

15-Minute Routine

(Beginner)

ORDER	EXERCISE	RESISTANCE/VARIATION	SETS
1	Squat	None	2
2	Squat Pulse	None	1
3	Dip	None	2
4	Jumpers	None	1
5	Squat and Lift	Eliminate lift	1
6	Bun Sweeps	None	1
7	Glute Raise	None	1

(Intermediate)

ORDER	EXERCISE	RESISTANCE/VARIATION	SETS
1	Squat	Dumbbells	2
2	Squat Pulse	None	1
3	Basic Lunge	None	2
4	Jumpers	None	1
5	Squat and Lift	None	1
6	Bun Sweeps	Pulse 8–12 times	1
7	Kneeling Glute Raise	Exercise band	1

(Advanced)

ORDER	EXERCISE	RESISTANCE/VARIATION	SETS
1	Squat	Dumbbells	2
2	Squat Pulse	Plié version	1
3	Basic Lunge	Dumbbells	2
4	Jumpers	None	1
5	Squat and Lift	None	1
6	Bun Sweeps	Ankle weight; pulse 8–12 times	1
7	Kneeling Glute Raise	Exercise band; pulse at top	1

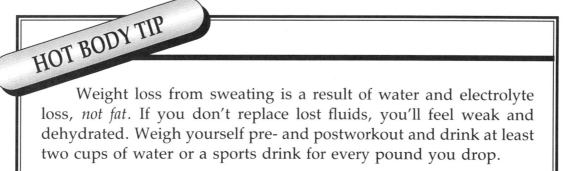

HOT BODY TIP

Weight loss from sweating is a result of water and electrolyte loss, *not fat*. If you don't replace lost fluids, you'll feel weak and dehydrated. Weigh yourself pre- and postworkout and drink at least two cups of water or a sports drink for every pound you drop.

20-Minute Routine

(Beginner)

ORDER	EXERCISE	RESISTANCE/VARIATION	SETS
1	Squat	None	2
2	Plié	None	1
3	Squat Pulse	None	1
4	Basic Lunge	None	2
5	Glute Raise	None	1
6	Squat and Lift	None	1
7	Bun Sweeps	None	2
8	Kneeling Glute Raise	Exercise band	1

(Intermediate)

ORDER	EXERCISE	RESISTANCE/VARIATION	SETS
1	Squat	Dumbbells	2
2	Plié	Dumbbell	1
3	Squat Pulse	None	1
4	Basic Lunge	None	2
5	3-D Lunge	None	1
6	Jumpers	None	1
7	Squat and Lift	None	1
8	Bun Sweeps	Ankle weight	1
9	Kneeling Glute Raise	Exercise band	1

(ADVANCED)

ORDER	EXERCISE	RESISTANCE/VARIATION	SETS
1	Squat	Dumbbells	2
2	Plié	Dumbbell	1
3	Squat Pulse	None	1
4	Basic Lunge	Dumbbells	2
5	3-D Lunge	None	1
6	Jumpers	None	1
7	Squat and Lift	None	1
8	Bun Sweeps	Ankle weight; pulse 8–12 times	1
9	Kneeling Glute Raise	Exercise band	1

HOT BODY TIP

If you simply can't resist a slice of cake, choose what will do the least damage: at 365 calories a slice, frosted devil's food cake is hell for your diet. Marble cake (270 calories) will weigh you down like bricks. Pound cake even sans icing packs a scale-tipping 200 calories per sliver. Your best bet is unadorned angel food cake at 140 calories per heavenly slice.

HOT BODY TIP

After a big meal, your body may tell you to take a walk. As usual, your body is right! Researchers have found that even moderate exercise an hour or so after eating helps more efficiently burn calories that might otherwise have wrapped around your waist.

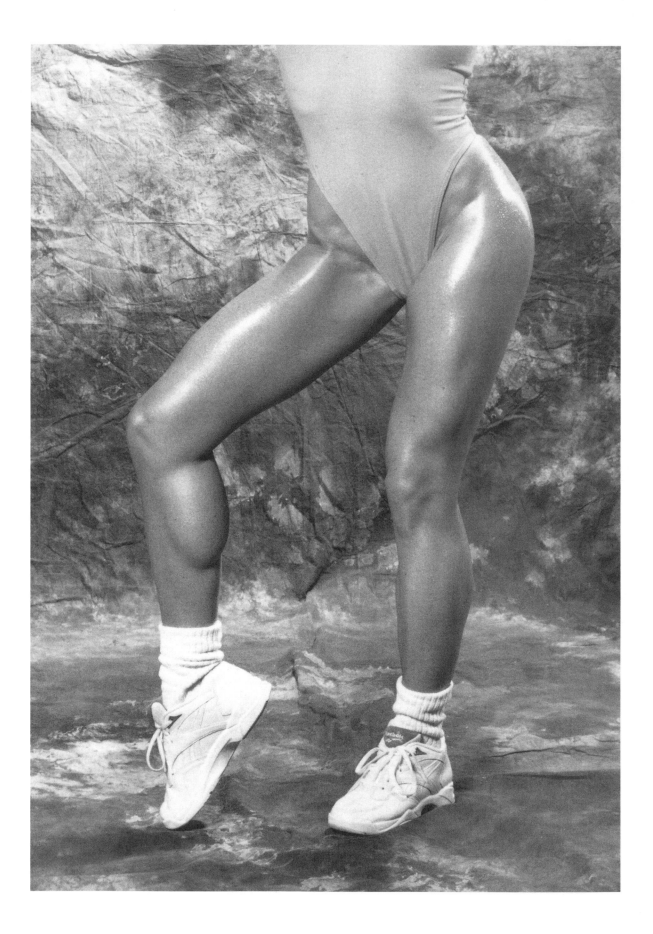

Inner and Outer Thighs

The most gorgeous set of buns will look even better if the inner and outer thighs form firm, tight curves. Since very few everyday activities—even most aerobic workouts, for that matter—work your inner and outer thighs to any great extent, target toning exercises are essential to firm up these muscles.

The Buns of Steel inner and outer thigh routine target tones these hard-to-reach muscles with laserlike precision. By doing the exercises in this chapter, you can expect the best inner and outer thighs you've ever had in your life. You'll love the results.

Several outer thigh muscles are also part of the buns. Consequently, when you isolate them and work them hard, don't be surprised if the shape of your buns also improves considerably. The exercises in this chapter are divided into target toners for your outer thighs and target toners for your inner thighs. To see the best improvements, work both muscle groups two to three times a week.

The great thing about working the outer thigh muscles is that it's easy to feel them working during target toning moves. And, with the help of the "Mind/Body Focus" tips, you'll know exactly what each move should feel like when you're doing it right. Outer thighs respond well to resistance training: in a little over a month you'll see definite results. You may find your inner thighs are a bit harder to feel when you're working them. If that's the case, concentrate on keeping your movements small and precise—you don't have to swing your leg all over the place to get these muscles into shape! It helps to pay attention to the "Mind/Body Focus" tips. With a little concentration and a lot of attention to technique, you'll see improvements in your inner thighs in just a few weeks.

The Inner and Outer Thigh Muscles

The inner and outer thigh muscles are known as your *leg adductors* and *abductors*, respectively. Have you ever noticed that figure skaters have outer thighs to die for? That's because, outside of target toning, skating is one of the few activities that really brings your outer thigh muscles into play. (By the way, skaters also do lots of target toning exercises for this area.)

You use your inner thigh muscles in activities like horseback riding. If you've ever been saddle sore after a day on horseback, you know where the muscles in your inner thighs are located! These newly toned inner thigh muscles will make a significant improvement in your appearance.

The eight exercises in this chapter help you focus on your inner and outer thighs. They are arranged into nine routines with varying time limits and fitness levels, so you can choose the one that is exactly right for *you*.

THIGH EXERCISES

Outer Thigh

1. Outward Step and Squat
2. Penguins
3. Hip Press
4. Side Lying Outward Rotation

Inner Thigh

5. Supported Inner Thigh Lift
6. Tilt and Squeeze
7. Glute Raise with Crossover
8. Inner Thigh Press-Out

HOT BODY TIP

There's nothing like a relaxing bubble bath, a soothing cup of herbal tea, or a leisurely walk around the block to clear your head, lower your blood pressure, and relieve that urge to binge on an entire bag of potato chips. Even a "breather"—closing your eyes and taking a few deep breaths—can be a pause that refreshes.

HOT BODY TIP

You've always thought that brown rice was much higher in fiber than white rice, but that's not the case. Half a cup of brown rice contains .2 gram of dietary fiber, while white rice is in the neighborhood of .1 gram. True, brown rice has slightly more protein, but it's also higher in calories—89 calories per half cup as opposed to 82 for white.

Outer Thigh

Exercise 1: OUTWARD STEP AND SQUAT

TARGET AREAS
Entire bun, hip, and thigh, with special emphasis on the outer hip and thigh.

The Setup: Place one or two sets of risers underneath your step. Stand next to the end of your step with your arms crossed at the wrists in front of you. Place your left foot on top of the step, keeping your right foot on the floor, bend both knees so that most of your weight is on your floor leg. Double-check your posture: stand tall with your shoulders relaxed, chest lifted, and abs tight.

The Move:
• Exhale. Press up off the ball of your right foot, point your toes, and straighten your right leg up and out to the side about six inches off the floor or until you feel the muscles in your outer hip contract. At the same time, bring your arms out to the sides until they are parallel to the floor.
• Inhale and return to the start. Land softly and roll your weight onto the heel of your floor foot.
• Switch legs and do the same number of reps.

Mind/Body Focus: Your landing on the downward movement should be soft and noiseless. You'll feel a contraction through your buns and both thighs as you press up, and you'll feel a strong pull through the outer hip of your working leg as it moves to the side.

Variations:
• If you find this move too difficult, do it without the step.
• If the arm movements throw you off, leave your arms at your sides.
• Curl your heel toward your buttocks as you reach the top of this movement to bring the back of the thigh into play.
• When you are ready for resistance, hold a dumbbell in each hand. When using dumbbells, hold your arms still, down at your sides.

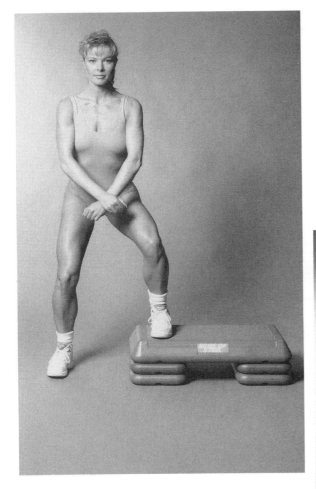

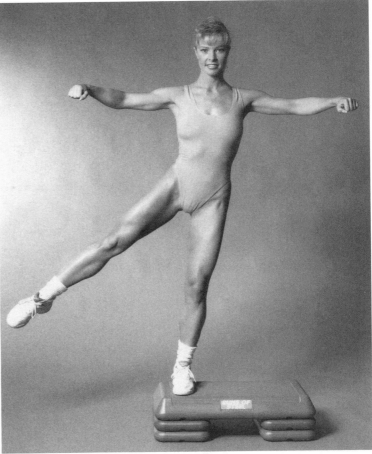

For Good Form and Safety:
- Keep both knees "soft" and springy to absorb the shock of each push-off and landing.
- Maintain good upper body posture so you don't fall forward.

Exercise 2: PENGUINS

TARGET AREAS
Works your outer hip and thigh.

The Setup: Stand with your feet hip width apart with an exercise band tied securely into a circle a few inches above your knees. Bend your knees slightly, and place your hands on your hips. Stand up tall and maintain a natural alignment.

The Move:
- Keeping both legs straight, exhale and lift your right leg up and out to the side about six inches, until the band is taut and you feel a contraction through your outer thigh.
- Hold for a moment at the top of the movement, and squeeze your buns together.
- Inhale and return your right foot to the floor.
- Repeat this movement with your left leg.
- Continue alternating legs. Do an equal number of reps on each side.

Mind/Body Focus: This exercise looks like a penguin waddling its way around the North Pole! You're doing it right if you feel continuous tension in your outer hips and thighs.

Variations:
- If you find this exercise too difficult, you may do it without the band. You may also hold on to a stable object placed in front of you for support.
- To add more resistance, make the band tighter or use a band with stronger tension.
- For a real outer thigh blaster, hold for a count of five at the top.

For Good Form and Safety:
- Once you feel the contraction in your outer thigh, there's no need to lift your leg any higher.
- Avoid arching your lower back, especially as you lift.

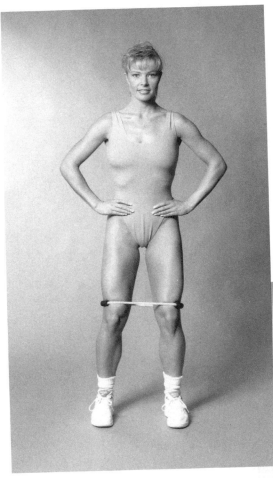

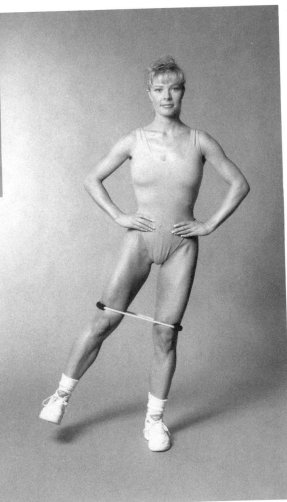

Exercise 3: HIP PRESS

TARGET AREAS
Isolates the outer thigh and the front of the thigh.

The Setup: Lie on one side on your exercise mat with your head resting on your outstretched arm. Bend your top arm and place that palm on the floor in front of your chest for support. Align your top hip directly over your bottom hip, and extend your bottom leg out straight; bend your top knee and rest it on the floor in front of your hip, with your foot flexed.

The Move:
- Exhale and lift your top leg up diagonally. In the finish position, your leg will be directly in line with your bottom leg and about six inches above it.
- Inhale and return your leg to the starting position.
- Lie on your other side, and do the same number of repetitions with your other leg.

Mind/Body Focus: Your setup is correct if there is a small space between your waist and the floor; maintain this space as you do this exercise. As you lift your leg imagine you are trying to press an object away from you with it: push and lift in one continuous movement. You'll feel a contraction in your outer hip and the front of your thigh as you lift.

Variations:
- For resistance, wrap a band around the arch of your working foot and the ankle of your base leg.
- To further zero in on your outer thigh, pulse up and down one to two inches, eight to twelve times at the top of the movement.

For Good Form and Safety:
- Don't roll your top hip backward as you do this exercise. To stabilize your body pull your abs inward and align your neck with the rest of your spine by tucking your chin.
- Don't arch your lower back, especially as you lift your leg.

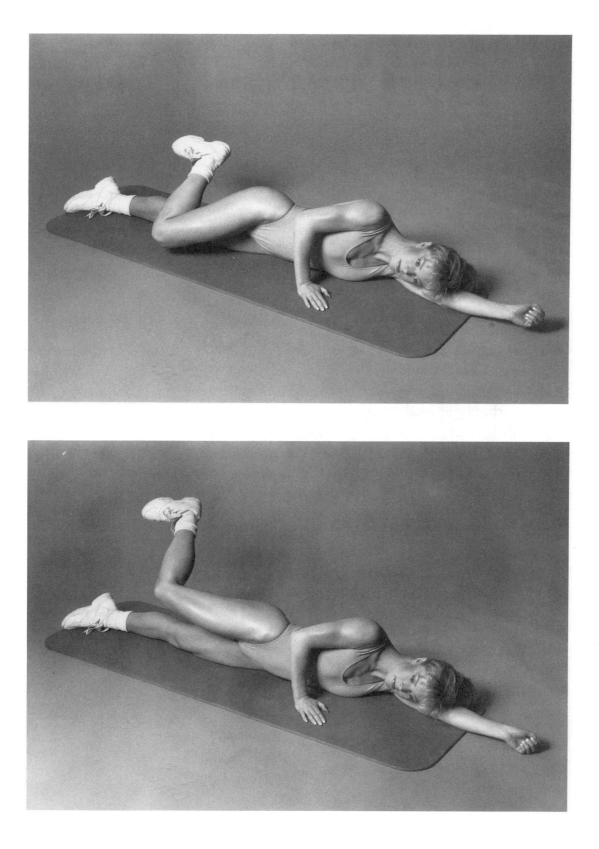

Exercise 4: SIDE LYING OUTWARD ROTATION

TARGET AREAS
Buns and outer hips and thighs.

The Setup: Lie on one side on your exercise mat with your head resting on your outstretched arm. Bend your top arm and place that palm on the floor in front of your chest for support. Align your top hip directly over your bottom hip. Bend your bottom knee slightly. Keeping your top leg slightly bent, flex your foot, lift your leg upward a few inches, and hold.

The Move:
• Inhale. Leading with your foot, turn your top leg in so that your toe is facing slightly downward.
• Exhale. Again leading with your foot, turn your top leg out so your toe is at a diagonal to the floor.
• Switch legs and do the same number of repetitions with the other leg.

Mind/Body Focus: Concentrate on lengthening your leg by pressing through your heel. Imagine you are trying to dig a hole in the dirt with it. When you're doing this exercise correctly you'll feel a contraction at the very top and outside of your outer hip as you point your foot upward.

Variations:
• For resistance, add an ankle weight.
• To make this exercise more advanced, hold in the outwardly rotated position and lift up and down.

For Good Form and Safety:
• Pull your abs inward and align your neck with the rest of your spine by tucking your chin. This will prevent you from rolling your hips backward and decreasing the effectiveness of the exercise.
• This is a *very small* movement. There's no need to exaggerate it to work the outer thigh.

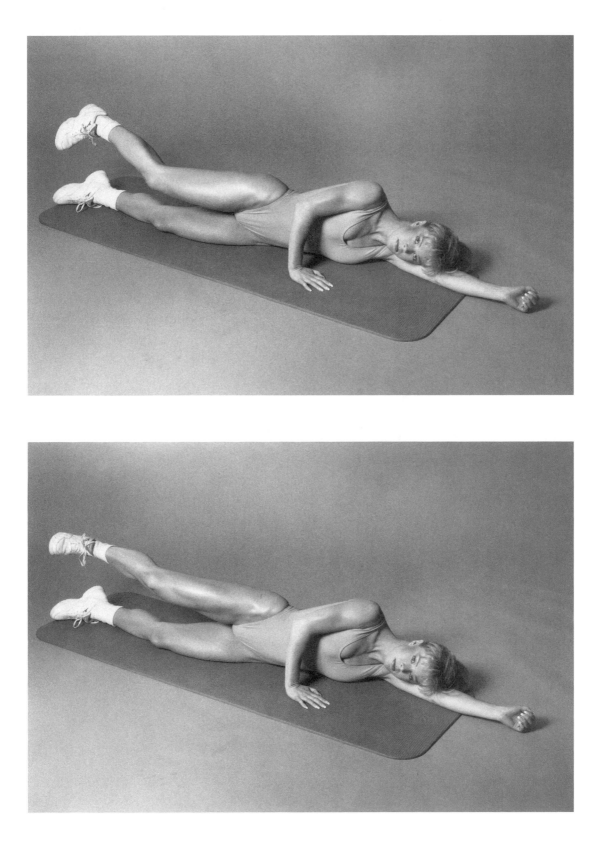

INNER THIGH

Exercise 5: SUPPORTED INNER THIGH LIFT

TARGET AREAS
This one blasts the inner thighs!

The Setup: Remove all risers from underneath your step. Lie on your left side behind the step. Extend your left arm and leg straight out and rest your head on your arm. Your top hip should be aligned directly over your bottom hip. Rest your right hand on top of the step for balance. Bend your right leg and rest it on top of the step so that your knee is in the center and your toe is resting on the bottom edge.

The Move:
- Exhale. Lengthen your bottom leg by extending through your heel, and lift it as high as you can.
- Pause briefly at the top of the movement, inhale, and slowly lower your leg back to the start.
- Switch sides and do an equal number of reps with the other leg.

Mind/Body Focus: Try to imagine a puppet string attached to your ankle gently pulling your leg upward and lowering it down again. You'll feel a strong contraction through the inner thigh of your working leg as you move upward and as you hold at the top.

Variations:
- For resistance, you may use an ankle weight or place a band around both ankles.
- More advanced exercisers may remove the step platform.

For Good Form and Safety:
- Don't roll back away from the bench as you move. Pulling your abdominals in and keeping your spine perfectly aligned will help you remain stable.

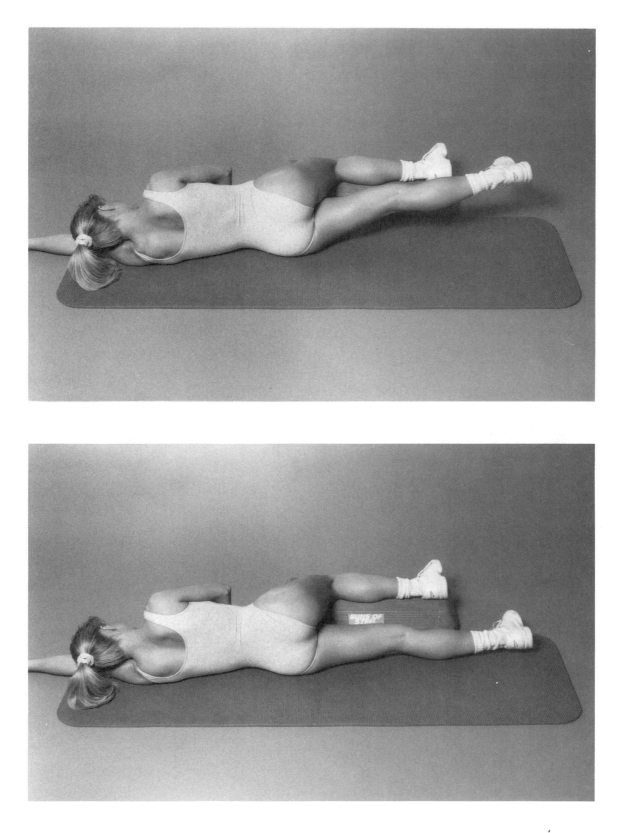

Exercise 6: TILT AND SQUEEZE

TARGET AREAS
Focuses on the buns, inner thighs, and backs of thighs. In addition, it's a terrific stretch for your lower back.

The Setup: Lie on your back on your mat with your arms behind your head or at your sides. Bend your knees and place your feet slightly apart and flat on the floor. Pull your abdominals in toward your spine and firmly anchor your lower back to the floor.

The Move:
- Squeeze your buttocks and tilt your pelvis upward so that your buns raise up off the floor *but your lower back remains firmly anchored*. Initiate the upward movement by pressing through your heels.
- At the top of the movement, exhale, and squeeze your knees together.
- Hold for a moment, inhale, and slowly lower to the start.

Mind/Body Focus: You should feel your back lengthening as your pelvis tilts upward. When you squeeze your thighs together, pretend you are trying to squeeze all the juice out of an orange. You're doing this exercise correctly if you feel your buns and the backs of your thighs working as you do the pelvic tilt and your inner thighs as you squeeze.

Variations:
- To make this exercise more challenging, try this "ball squeeze" version: Place a tennis ball, rolled-up towel, or weighted exercise ball between your knees. Give it a good squeeze so you don't drop it as you move through the exercise.
- To increase the intensity, hold at the top and continue squeezing for a slow count of five.
- Another way to make this move more challenging is to pulse your pelvis a very small way up and down eight to twelve times, one to two inches in the topmost position.

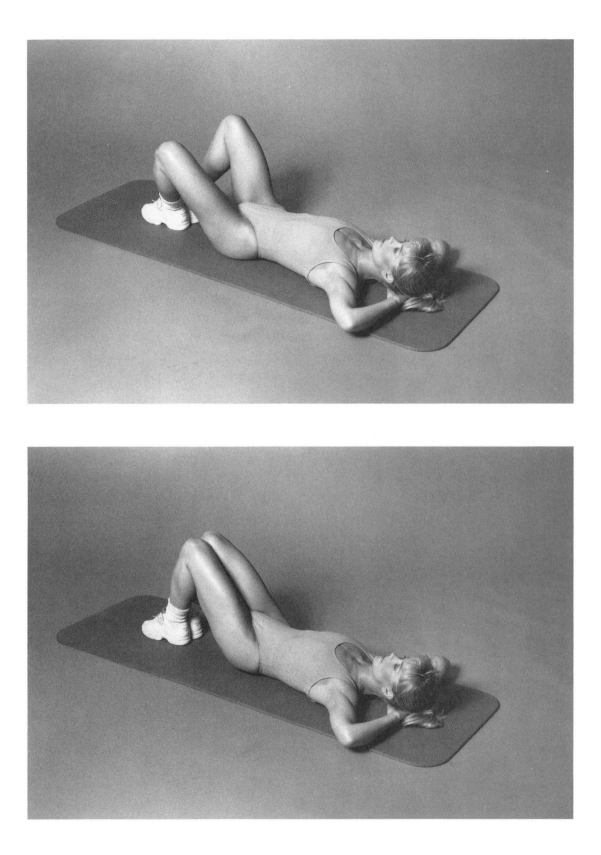

Exercise 7: GLUTE RAISE WITH CROSSOVER

TARGET AREAS
Buns and back of thigh, with special emphasis on the inner thigh.

The Setup: Kneel on your knees and elbows with your weight distributed as evenly as possible. Your elbows should be directly under your shoulders. Align your neck with the rest of your spine by tucking your chin in slightly.

The Move:
- Exhale. With a flexed foot, keeping your knee bent in a 90-degree angle, lift one knee up to hip height so that the sole of your foot is pressed up toward the ceiling.
- Inhale. Keeping your knee bent, lower your leg and, as you do so, cross your knee over to the outside of the calf of your other leg.
- Lower your knee so that it's just off the floor.
- Do an equal number of reps with the other leg.

Mind/Body Focus: You'll feel the muscles in your buns and the back of the working thigh contract as you press upward; as you cross over, you'll feel tension in both of your inner thighs.

Variations:
- For resistance, add an ankle weight.
- To add more bun work, alternate one crossover with one press straight upward.
- If you find this exercise difficult, lower your knee halfway.

For Good Form and Safety:
- Don't allow your knee to travel higher than hip level!
- In order to keep your balance and prevent your lower back from sagging downward, pull your abdominals in toward your spine.

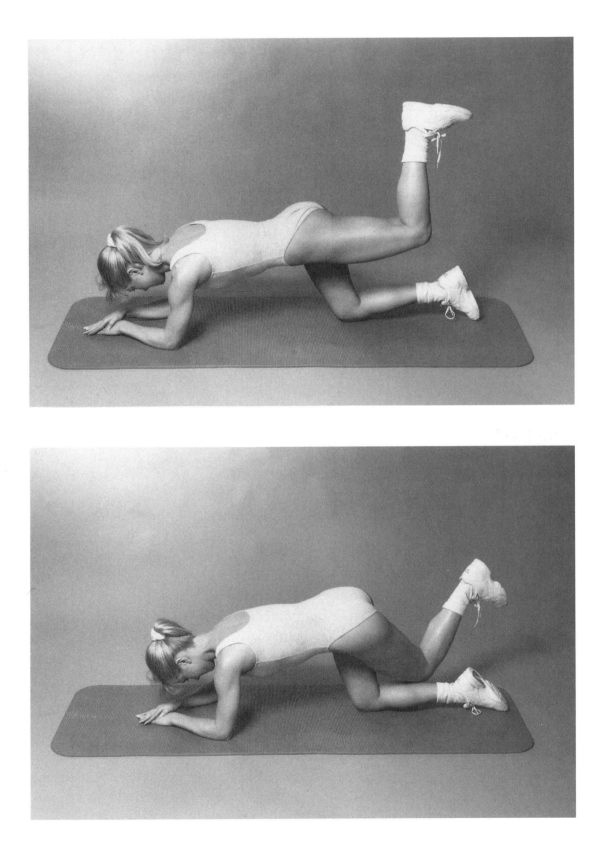

Exercise 8: INNER THIGH PRESS-OUT

TARGET AREAS

Isolates the inner thighs. An added bonus: you'll strengthen your arms and chest, too!

The Setup: Lie on your back on your mat with your arms at your sides. Spread your legs a few feet apart and straighten them upward so that they are directly over your hips. Flex your feet so your soles are facing the ceiling. Cross one arm over the other and place the palm of each hand on the inside of the opposite thigh below the knee.

The Move:
- Exhale. Close your legs together while resisting the inward movement by pressing outward with your hands. Do this for a slow count of five, taking care to maintain proper alignment.
- Inhale. Return to the start.

Mind/Body Focus:

Imagine your thighs are two walls that are closing in and you must resist them with your hands. You're doing this right if you feel pressure on your inner thighs from the tops of your legs to the insides of your knees as you resist inward. Additionally, you'll feel your arms and chest working.

Variations:
- For a very intense inner thigh workout, allow your arms and legs to resist each other in both directions. As you move your legs back to the start, push outward with your hands as you move inward with your thighs.
- If you find this exercise too difficult, do it without your arms for resistance.
- If you want to add outer thigh to this movement, place an exercise band around your thighs just above your knees.

For Good Form and Safety:
- If you aren't flexible enough to straighten your legs completely, it's okay to bend your knees as much as you need.
- *Keep your back firmly in contact with your mat throughout the entire exercise.* Pull your abdominals inward and anchor your entire spine to the floor.

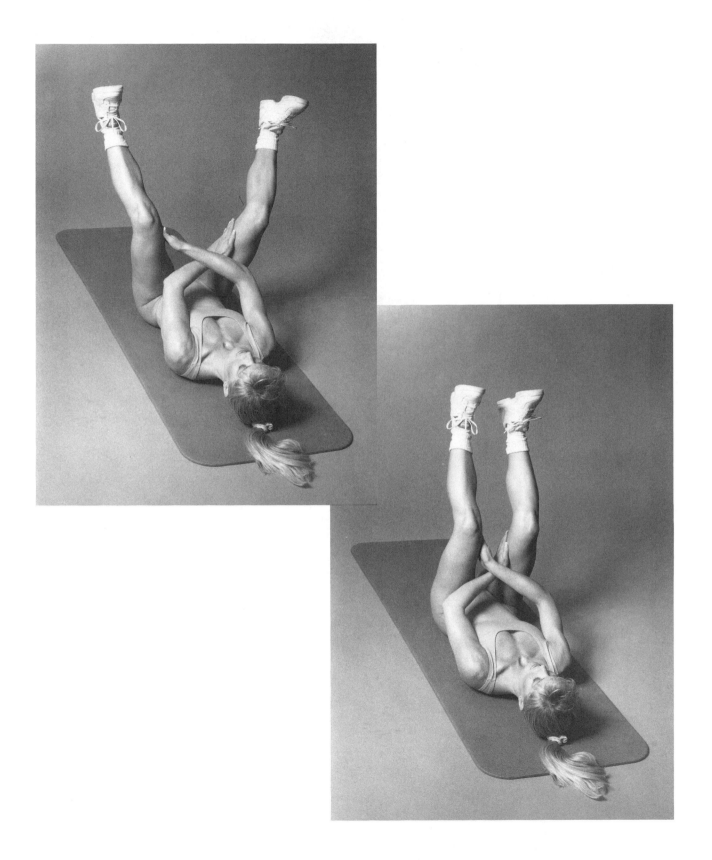

Inner and Outer Thigh Routines

Here are three inner/outer thigh routines you can try. Figure out how much time you want to spend target toning this area (ten, fifteen, or twenty minutes), then adapt that routine to your level. Once you've tried our routines for a while, mix and match the exercises to make up routines of your own.

Equipment you'll need: A step, exercise band or tube, and mat.

Optional for variations: One or two sets of risers, one or more sets of dumbbells, one or more ankle weights, tennis or weighted ball.

How Many Reps Should I Do?

Contrary to what you may have learned in the past, doing hundreds and hundreds of leg lifts while lying on your side is not a very good way to target tone this area. It's not only time-consuming, it's boring and ineffective. Do eight to fifteen repetitions of each set of inner and outer thigh exercises. When you can do fifteen repetitions easily and with good form, move on to a more difficult variation of that exercise the next time you work out. If you find it difficult to do at least eight repetitions while maintaining good form, try an easier version of the exercise.

How Much Weight Should I Use?

When using resistance (dumbbell, ankle weight, or exercise band), choose a weight that will allow you to complete eight to fifteen repetitions with proper form. Increase the weight when you can do fifteen reps easily and with good form; if you can't get through at least eight reps, decrease the weight.

Beginners, when you first try an exercise it will probably be challenging enough without adding dumbbells or using an ankle weight. When you're ready to add resistance, start with three- to five-pound dumbbells or, when called for, a one- to two-pound ankle weight. Always use an exercise band if it's included in the description of the basic version of an exercise. Intermediates, you'll use five- to ten-pound weights for most exercises and a two- to three-pound ankle weight. Advanced target toners, start with eight- to twelve-pound dumbbells and a three- to five-pound ankle weight. Of course, these recommendations are only guidelines—the weight you use should make the exercise more challenging, but you should still be able to maintain good form.

How Much Should I Rest Between Sets?

Rest from thirty to ninety seconds between each exercise set. This will allow your muscles enough time to recover so they are strong enough to work their hardest when you do the next set but will not be so long that you lose the intensity and focus of your workout. You'll find that as you become stronger you won't need to rest as much between sets.

How Often Should I Target Tone My Inner and Outer Thighs?

For best results, target tone your inner and outer thighs three times a week with at least one day of rest in between each workout session.

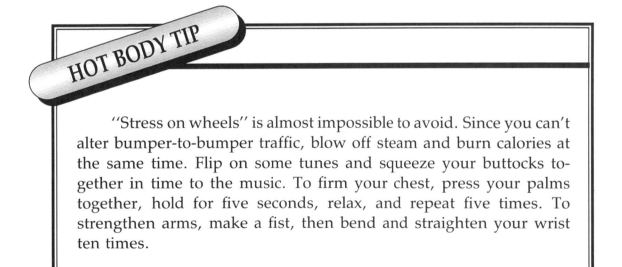

HOT BODY TIP

"Stress on wheels" is almost impossible to avoid. Since you can't alter bumper-to-bumper traffic, blow off steam and burn calories at the same time. Flip on some tunes and squeeze your buttocks together in time to the music. To firm your chest, press your palms together, hold for five seconds, relax, and repeat five times. To strengthen arms, make a fist, then bend and straighten your wrist ten times.

Thigh Isolation Routines
10-Minute Routines
(Beginner)

ORDER	EXERCISE	RESISTANCE	SETS
1	Hip Press	None	1
2	Outward Rotation	None	2
3	Penguins	Exercise band	1
4	Tilt and Squeeze	None	1
5	Supported Inner Thigh Lift	None	1
6	Glute Raise with Crossover	None	1

(Intermediate)

ORDER	EXERCISE	RESISTANCE	SETS
1	Hip Press	Exercise band	1
2	Outward Rotation	None	2
3	Penguins	Exercise band	1
4	Tilt and Squeeze	Ball squeeze version (pg. 102)	1
5	Supported Inner Thigh Lift	Exercise band	1
6	Glute Raise with Crossover	None	1

(Advanced)

ORDER	EXERCISE	RESISTANCE	SETS
1	Hip Press	Exercise band; pulse at top	1
2	Outward Rotation	None	2
3	Penguins	Exercise band	1
4	Tilt and Squeeze	Ball squeeze version (pg. 102); 5-second hold	1
5	Supported Inner Thigh Lift	Exercise band	1
6	Glute Raise with Crossover	None	1

15-MINUTE ROUTINE

(BEGINNER)

ORDER	EXERCISE	RESISTANCE/VARIATION	SETS
1	Hip Press	None	2
2	Penguins	Exercise band	1
3	Outward Rotation	None	2
4	Tilt and Squeeze	None	1
5	Supported Inner Thigh Lift	None	1
6	Glute Raise with Crossover	None	1
7	Inner Thigh Press-Out	None	1

(INTERMEDIATE)

ORDER	EXERCISE	RESISTANCE/VARIATION	SETS
1	Hip Press	Exercise band	2
2	Penguins	Exercise band	1
3	Outward Rotation	None	1
4	Outward Step and Squat	None	1
5	Tilt and Squeeze	Ball squeeze version (pg. 102)	1
6	Supported Inner Thigh Lift	None	1
7	Glute Raise with Crossover	Alternate with Glute Raise	1
8	Inner Thigh Press-Out	None	1

(Advanced)

ORDER	EXERCISE	RESISTANCE/VARIATION	SETS
1	Hip Press	Exercise band	2
2	Penguins	Exercise band	1
3	Outward Rotation	Ankle weight	1
4	Outward Step and Squat	Dumbbells	1
5	Tilt and Squeeze	Ball squeeze version (pg. 102); 5-second hold	1
6	Supported Inner Thigh Lift	Exercise band	1
7	Glute Raise with Crossover	Alternate with Glute Raise	1
8	Inner Thigh Press-Out	None	1

20-Minute Routine

(Beginner)

ORDER	EXERCISE	RESISTANCE/VARIATION	SETS
1	Hip Press	None	2
2	Penguins	Exercise band	1
3	Outward Rotation	None	2
4	Outward Step and Squat	None	2
5	Tilt and Squeeze	None	1
6	Supported Inner Thigh Lift	None	2
7	Glute Raise with Crossover	None	1
8	Inner Thigh Press-Out	None	2

(INTERMEDIATE)

ORDER	EXERCISE	RESISTANCE/VARIATION	SETS
1	Hip Press	Ankle weight	2
2	Penguins	Exercise band	1
3	Outward Rotation	Ankle weight	2
4	Outward Step and Squat	Add leg curls	2
5	Tilt and Squeeze	Ball squeeze version (pg. 102); 5-second hold	1
6	Supported Inner Thigh Lift	Exercise band	2
7	Glute Raise with Crossover	Alternate with Glute Raise	1
8	Inner Thigh Press-Out	None	2

(ADVANCED)

ORDER	EXERCISE	RESISTANCE/VARIATION	SETS
1	Hip Press	Ankle weight; pulse 12 times at top	2
2	Penguins	Exercise band	1
3	Outward Rotation	Ankle weight; lift and lower in rotated position	2
4	Outward Step and Squat	Dumbbells; add leg curls	2
5	Tilt and Squeeze	Ball squeeze version (pg. 102); 5-second hold	1
6	Supported Inner Thigh Lift	Exercise band; remove step	2
7	Glute Raise with Crossover	Alternate with Glute Raise	1
8	Inner Thigh Press-Out	None	2

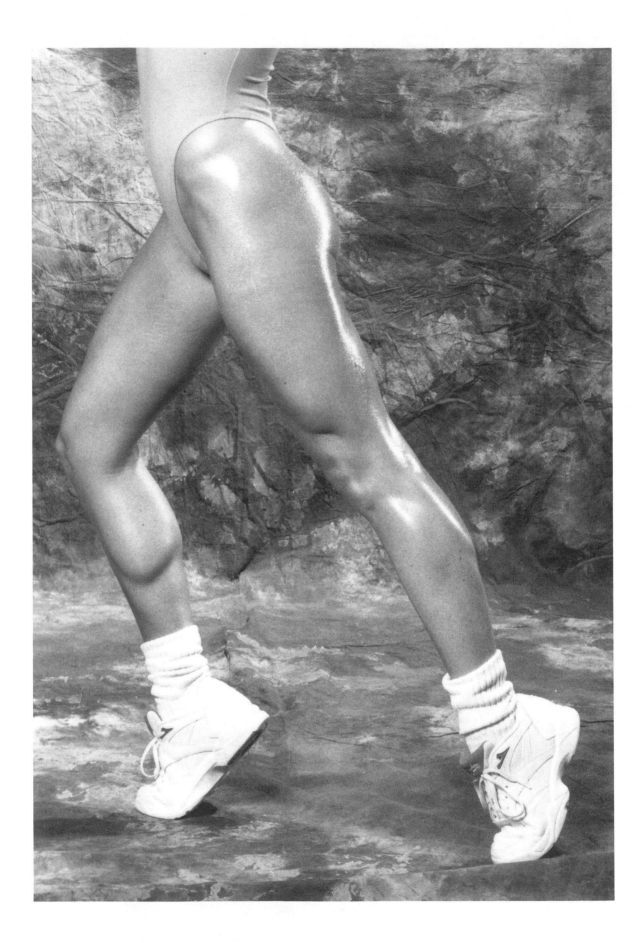

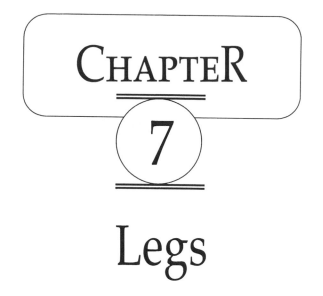

Legs

Picture this: a pair of beautifully toned thighs that taper into sculpted, shapely calves. Now picture this: those legs belong to you. Impossible, you say? Well, it's not. The exercises we've selected for this chapter are designed to make a difference. A difference anyone will see if they do them faithfully. No matter what size or shape your legs are, the Buns of Steel legs routine can help you create legs that you'll be proud to display in short shorts, minis, and even French-cut bikinis. Your thighs will be lean and muscular in the front, with a defined, sleek sweep in the back. Your curvaceous lower legs will make heads turn. Before you know it, you'll be raising the hems on your skirts to show off the results!

Because the muscles in the front of the thigh are relatively easy to isolate, you'll really feel them as you exercise. As these muscles grow stronger you'll begin to notice definition, or "muscularity." When they're firm and toned they'll actually seem longer, too. With consistent training, the back of your thigh will also develop definition. You may feel the exercises for the backs of your thighs more than the front of the thigh target toners during the first couple of workouts because they're normally not as strong as the fronts of the thighs. But since they respond so readily to target toning exercises, you'll notice significant improvements after just a few workouts.

As for calves, everyone has different genetics: some people have long calf muscles that run from the bottom of their knee to the top of their heel; others have short, high muscles that stop in the middle of their lower leg. However, any well-trained calf muscle will always have a distinctive curve and a well-toned, muscular appearance.

Most people will see noticeable results in their legs in about six weeks if they work them consistently three times a week.

The Leg Muscles

You really depend on the *quadriceps*, as the four muscles in the front of your thigh are known. They're the main muscles you use when you walk, run, bike, sit, stand—just about any movement you make with your legs. You rely on the muscles in the back of your thigh, the *hamstrings*, to balance the actions of your "quads." Your *calf* muscles give shape to the back of your lower legs; you use them every time you jump up to catch a ball or stand up on your tiptoes to reach something on the top shelf.

In this chapter you will find nine exercises for your legs, with individualized routines to give you the workout that's right for *your* front and back thighs and calves.

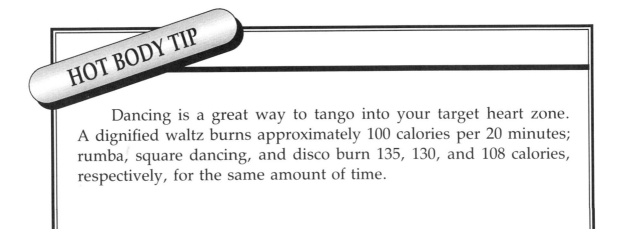

HOT BODY TIP

Dancing is a great way to tango into your target heart zone. A dignified waltz burns approximately 100 calories per 20 minutes; rumba, square dancing, and disco burn 135, 130, and 108 calories, respectively, for the same amount of time.

Leg Exercises

Front of Thigh

1. Wall Sit
2. One Leg Quad Pulse
3. Standing Leg Extension with Band
4. Bump Squat

Back of Thigh

5. Step and Curl
6. Standing Leg Curl with Band
7. Kneeling Four-Count Leg Curl

Calf

8. Standing Calf Raise Off Step
9. Seated Calf Raise

HOT BODY TIP

Turn today's trip to the mall into a workout. You'll burn eleven calories per minute if you forgo the elevator and take the stairs instead—and up to sixteen calories per minute if you take them in a hurry. (Just be sure to wear cushioned athletic shoes and hold on to the handrail.) If you're riding up an escalator, hold on to the rail and let your heels hang off the edge of the step, an effective stretch for tired, shopped-out calf muscles. And check your local Yellow Pages to see if your mall has a mall walkers club that meets before opening so you can mix a little window-shopping with your exercise.

FRONT OF THIGH

Exercise 1: WALL SIT

TARGET AREAS

Skiers and skaters use this exercise to target tone the fronts of their thighs. Bonus: improves posture.

The Setup: Stand with your back against a wall with your arms extended out in front of you at shoulder height and your feet about a foot away from the wall and flat on the floor. Maintain good posture by keeping your spine aligned naturally, your shoulders relaxed, and your abdominals pulled inward. Keep your neck in line with your spine.

The Move:

- Slide your body down along the wall, stopping when your hips are a few inches above your knees.
- Hold this position for fifteen seconds as you concentrate on your body's alignment.
- Slide up to the start.
- This is one repetition; three repetitions of this exercise is a set.

Mind/Body Focus: You are in the correct setup position if there is a very slight gap between the small of your back and the wall. In the down position, pretend you're sitting on an imaginary chair. You'll immediately feel tension in the tops of your thighs as you move into the seated position; this tension will grow stronger as you hold the repetition.

Variations:

- If you can't hold the seated position for fifteen seconds, do it for five seconds.
- To make this exercise more challenging: lower till your knees are in line with your hips.
- To advance, gradually increase your hold time to forty-five seconds.
- For the ultimate thigh target toner, try this "wall slide" version: Go into the seated position and, instead of holding, slide up and down a few inches for eight to twelve repetitions.

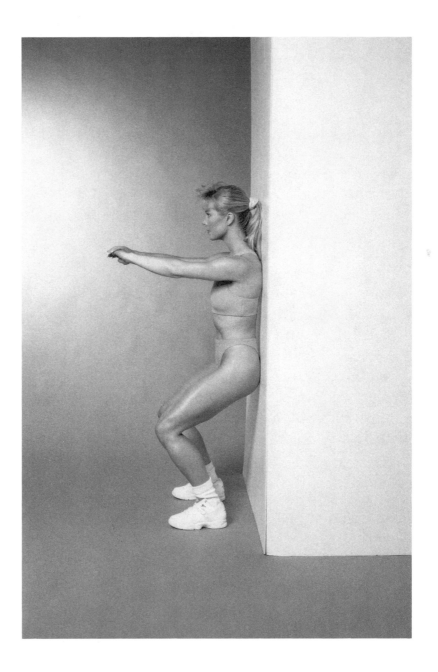

For Good Form and Safety:

- *Don't allow your knees to move forward of your toes.* You can avoid this by making sure your hips don't drop lower than knee level.
- If you have high blood pressure, limit your wall sit time to ten seconds and under.
- It's essential to keep breathing during this exercise. Don't hold your breath!

119

Exercise 2: ONE LEG QUAD PULSE

TARGET AREAS
Works the front of the thigh as well as the back of the thigh and buns.

The Setup: Stand an arm's length away from a stable object such as a sturdy chair; hold on to it for support. Stand on your left leg and tuck your right ankle behind your left ankle, with your right foot an inch off the floor.

The Move:
- Inhale. While maintaining good posture, bend your left knee and lower your body a few inches toward the floor.
- Exhale. Return to the start.
- Switch legs, and do an equal number of repetitions.

Mind/Body Focus: To get the most from this exercise do it slowly: move down for a two-second count and then up for a two-second count. You're doing it right when you feel the muscles in the front of your thigh contracting both on the way up and the way down.

Variations:
- If you find this exercise too easy, you can increase the range of motion by lowering your working leg into a squat position (thigh parallel to the floor).
- To add resistance, hold a dumbbell in the hand on the opposite side of your standing leg.

For Good Form and Safety:
- Good posture will increase the effectiveness of this exercise, so be sure to stand up tall and pull in your abs.
- Don't "lock" or fully straighten your knee as you move back up to the standing position.

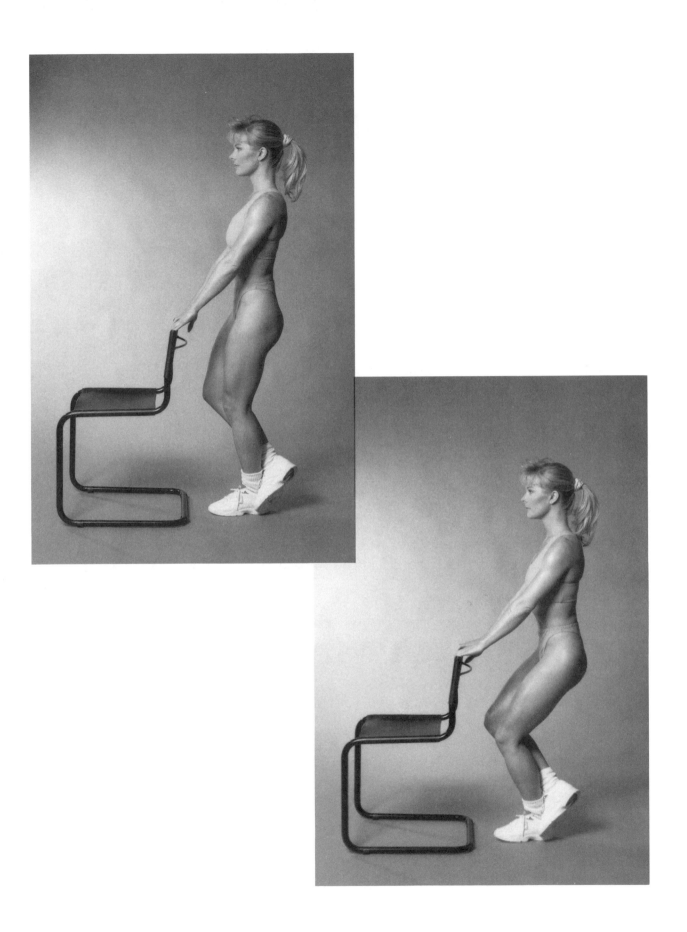

121

Exercise 3: STANDING LEG EXTENSION WITH BAND

TARGET AREAS
Isolates the front of your thigh.

The Setup: Tie together two ends of about two feet of an exercise band or tube; make sure the knot is secure. Place this "band circle" around both ankles. Stand on your right leg. Bend your left knee and lift it till your foot is in front of you and level with the middle of your right calf; flex your left foot so that the sole is facing the floor. You may hold on to a stable object at your side to help you keep your balance.

The Move:
- Exhale. Leading with your heel, straighten your left leg out in front of you. At the top of the movement the band will be taut.
- Inhale and return to the starting position.
- Switch legs, and do the same number of repetitions.

Mind/Body Focus: Pretend you're kicking a ball slowly away from you as you straighten your leg. You'll feel the muscles in the front of your thigh working as it extends.

Variations:
- At the top of the movement, pulse up and down one to two inches before lowering.
- If you find this move too difficult to do standing, you can do it seated.

For Good Form and Safety:
- Don't fully straighten your knee. Keep it "soft" in the extended position.

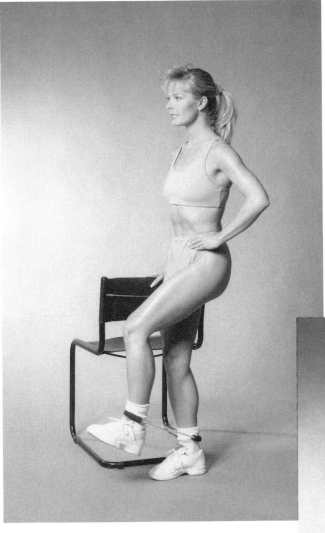

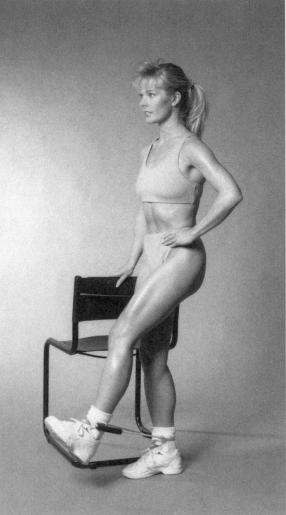

Exercise 4: BUMP SQUAT

TARGET AREAS

The ultimate front of thigh target toner! Works the buns and the back of thigh, too.

The Setup: Face a stable object such as a sturdy pole, door, or bedpost and, standing an arm's length away, hold your arms up at waist level and grasp it with both hands for support. Stand with your feet hip width apart and your toes facing forward.

The Move:
• Inhale and sit backward and downward until your thighs are parallel to the floor.
• Exhale. Squeeze your buns together and thrust your hips forward as you raise your body upward by straightening your legs. In the topmost position you'll be leaning backward at about a 30-degree angle and your knees will still be slightly bent. Your feet should remain flat on the floor throughout the movement.
• Return to the seated position by sitting straight downward from the leaning position.

Mind/Body Focus: The hip thrust in this exercise is like doing "the bump and grind." Don't put an excessive amount of force into this thrust; instead, concentrate on squeezing your buns and tightening the fronts of your thighs as you move upward. You'll feel this in the fronts of your thighs, your buns, and down the backs of your thighs as you move into the lean, especially as you reach the very top of the movement, and you'll feel the fronts of your thighs stretching as you lower your body into the sit.

Variations:
• For a real challenge, do this move while standing on tiptoe.
• Avoid "rolling" your hips from one position to the next.

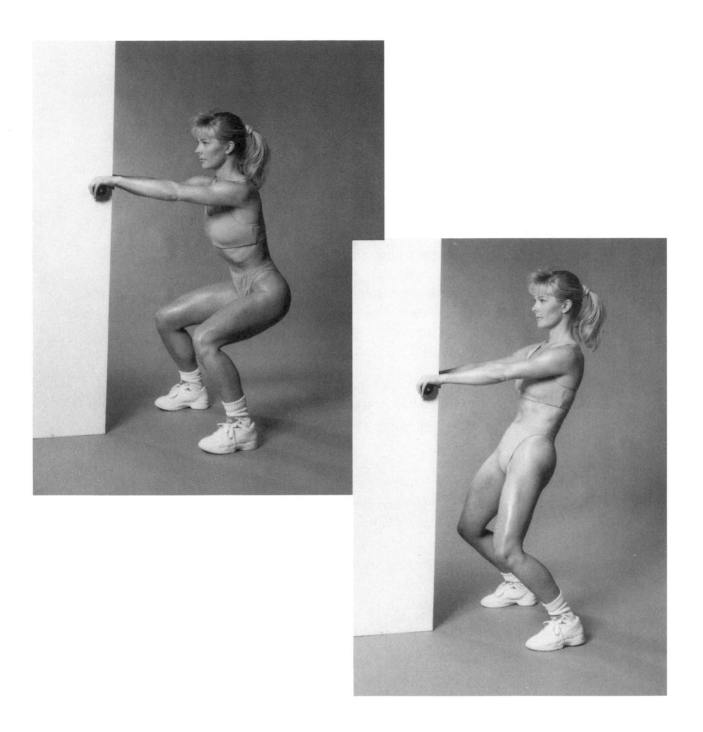

For Good Form and Safety:
- To prevent your lower back from overarching, good posture is important: stand tall, pull your abdominals inward, and maintain a natural arch in your spine.
- Pay attention to knee positioning as you move through this exercise! Don't allow your knees to move forward of your toes as you sit down, and don't fully straighten them when you move upward.

125

Back of Thigh

Exercise 5: STEP AND CURL

TARGET AREAS
Target tones the back of the thigh, front of the thigh, and buns.

The Setup: Stand with your step in front of you. Rest your right foot lightly on top of it; have both knees slightly bent. Most of your weight should be on your left leg. Leave your hands at your sides and stand up tall by relaxing your shoulders and pulling your abdominals inward.

The Move:
- Exhale. Roll your weight onto your right foot and step up onto the step. Lean slightly forward, and lift your left foot off the floor by bending your knee behind you.
- Continue bending your knee, curling your heel up toward your buns. In the topmost position your left heel will be a few inches above knee level, with your knee pointing toward the floor.
- Inhale and return to the start. When you return your left foot to the floor, land softly on the ball of your foot and roll through to your heel.
- Curl both arms up toward your shoulders as you step up, and press them backward as you lower.
- Switch legs and do an equal number of reps.

Mind/Body Focus: Imagine your working leg as a nutcracker, and try to crack a walnut as you bend your knee. You'll feel this move in the front thigh of your base leg as you press up and the back thigh of your working leg as you curl.

Variations:
- If you find this exercise too difficult, do it without the step.
- To add resistance, hold a dumbbell in each hand.

For Good Form and Safety:
- Don't allow the knee of your curling leg to come forward of your base leg.
- Keep both of your knees "soft."

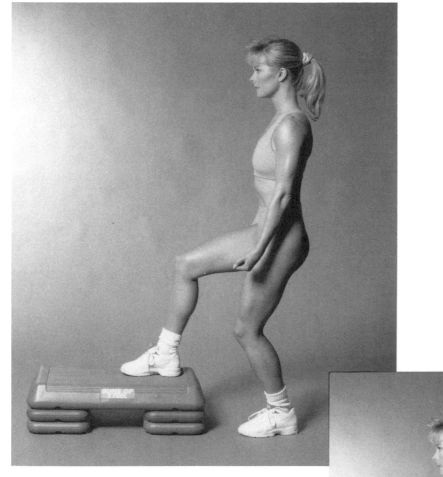
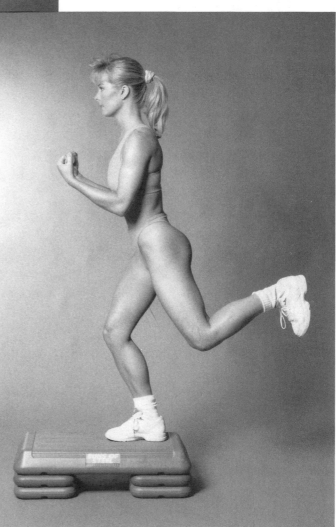

Exercise 6: STANDING LEG CURL WITH BAND

TARGET AREAS
Isolates the back of the thigh.

The Setup: Tie together the two ends of about two feet of an exercise band or tube; make sure the knot is secure. Place this "band circle" around your ankles. Stand on your right foot. Keeping your left knee slightly bent, extend your left leg behind you so that your foot comes off the floor about six inches and there is a slight tension on the band. You may hold on to a stable object for balance, or place your hands on your hips.

The Move:
- Flex your left foot. Exhale and curl your heel upward toward your buttocks. In the topmost position your knee will be bent at a 90-degree angle.
- Inhale and lower your leg to the start.
- Switch legs and do an equal number of reps.

Mind/Body Focus: As with all leg curl moves, pretend you have a nut behind your knee that you're trying to crack. You'll feel the muscles in the back of your thigh contract as you curl your leg toward your buttocks.

Variations:
- To increase resistance, tighten the band or switch to a stronger band.
- If you find this move too difficult, you can do it without a band.
- To make this move more challenging, at the top of the movement pulse up and down one to two inches before uncurling your leg.

For Good Form and Safety:
- Don't allow the knee of your curling leg to move forward of your base leg.
- Standing tall with good posture will increase the effectiveness of this exercise.

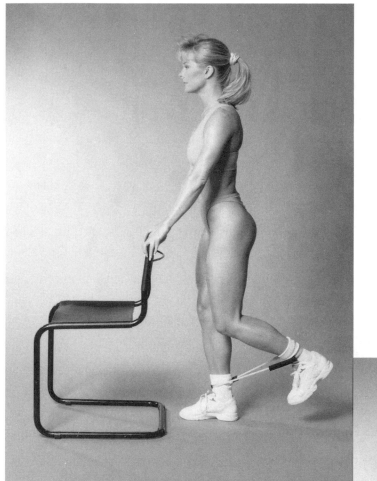

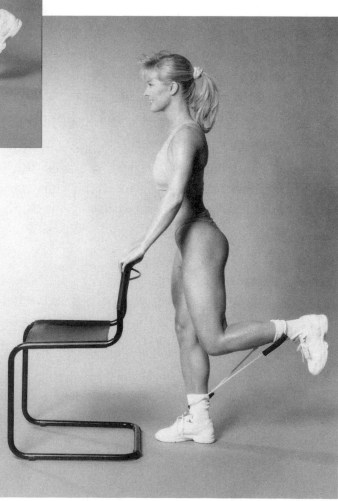

Exercise 7: KNEELING FOUR-COUNT LEG CURL

TARGET AREAS
Back of thigh and buns.

The Setup: Kneel on your knees and elbows with your weight distributed as evenly as possible. Align your neck with the rest of your spine by tucking your chin in slightly.

The Move:
- Exhale. Squeeze your buns together, flex your left foot and, keeping your left knee bent, lift it off the floor until the back of your thigh is parallel to the floor and the sole of your foot is facing directly up toward the ceiling.
- Inhale and, leading with your heel, straighten your leg out behind you.
- Exhale, bend your knee, and begin curling your leg back to the first position.
- Inhale and lower to the start.
- Switch legs and do an equal number of repetitions.

Mind/Body Focus: Every phase of this exercise is connected to the other phases. Done correctly, it requires only a brief pause as you move from one position to the next so that it has a smooth, continuous feel. You'll feel tension in your buns and back of thigh as you lift your leg; the tension in the back of your thigh will increase when you curl your leg back to position one.

Variations:
- To add resistance, you may place a band underneath the top of your right foot and around the arch of your left foot.
- To completely isolate the back of the thigh, curl and straighten your up-lifted leg eight to twelve times.

For Good Form and Safety:
- To prevent your lower back from sagging downward, pull your abdominals in toward your spine and allow your spine to maintain a natural curve.
- Don't "fly" through this exercise by using jerky knee movements.
- Your thigh should never move above hip level.

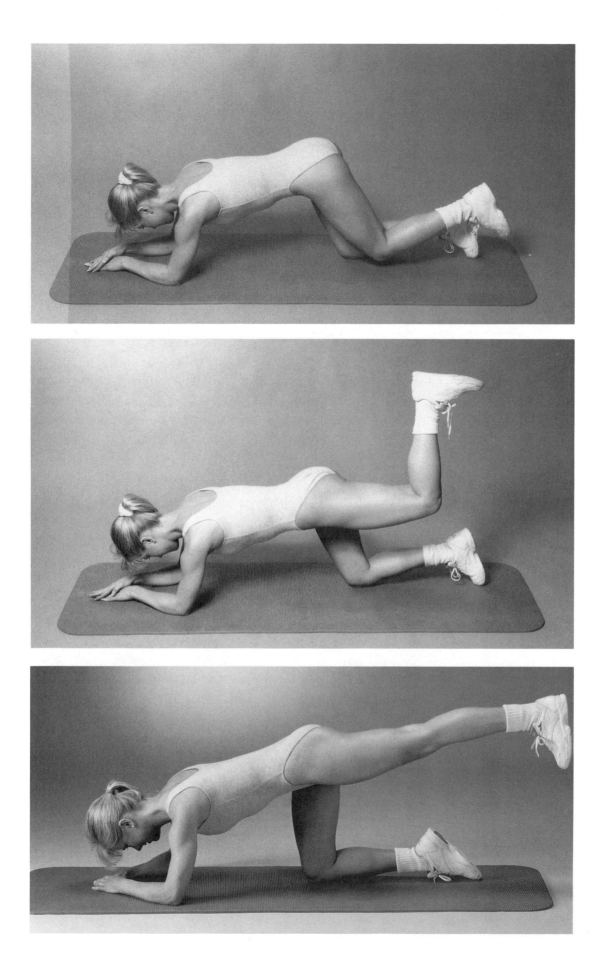

Calf

Exercise 8: STANDING CALF RAISE OFF STEP

TARGET AREAS
Target tones the back of the lower leg (calf).

The Setup: For this exercise you'll need a step that's at least four inches high. Hold on to a stable object placed beside you and stand on the end of the step with your feet hip width apart. Place the balls of your feet on the edge of the step so that your heels are hanging off. Stand up tall, and maintain a natural curve in your spine.

The Move:
- Exhale. Raise up on your tiptoes as high as you can go.
- Hold for a moment at the top of the movement, then inhale and lower your heels below the top of the step.

Mind/Body Focus: Pretend you're trying to peek over a fence. You'll feel a strong tension in your calf as you raise upward and a stretch through your calf when you lower your heels below the step.

Variations:
- To add resistance, hold a dumbbell in one hand with your arm either down at your side or your elbow bent with the weight resting on your shoulder.
- To isolate one leg at a time, you can do a one-leg calf raise: wrap one foot behind your other ankle and lift and lower with your base leg. Do an equal number of reps with both legs.
- At the top of the movement, pulse up and down one to two inches, eight to twelve times before lowering.

Good Form and Safety:
- It's okay to keep your knees fully straightened because they're not "involved" in the movement, but don't completely lock your knees.

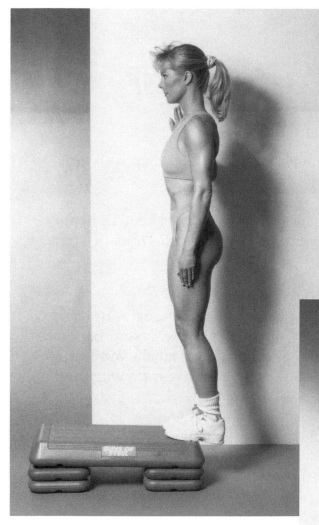

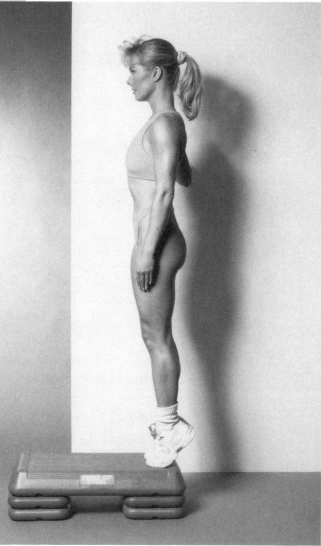

133

Exercise 9: SEATED CALF RAISE

TARGET AREAS
Works the back of your lower leg (calf). Bonus: you'll strengthen your arms as well.

The Setup: Sit up tall on the edge of a chair with your knees bent and your feet flat on the floor. Place the heels of your hands on the tops of your thighs.

The Move:
- Exhale. Raise up on your tiptoes as high as you can go. Resist this upward movement by pushing down on the tops of your thighs with your hands.
- Hold for a moment at the top of the movement, then inhale and lower slowly to the start, maintaining a constant downward pressure with your hands.

Mind/Body Focus: As you're raising your heels, imagine you're trying to close a suitcase that doesn't want to close—it seems the more you push down, the more it wants to pop up! You'll feel a contraction deep and in the center of your calves as you move upward; this will be especially intense as you hold at the top of the movement.

Variations:
- To increase the range of motion, place the balls of your feet on the edge of your step so that your heels are hanging off. When you lower let your heels travel below the level of the step.
- To increase resistance, hold a dumbbell on your thighs.
- To isolate one leg at a time, you can do a one-leg calf raise: wrap one foot behind your other ankle and lift and lower with your base leg. Do an equal number of reps with both legs.
- At the top of the movement, pulse up and down one to two inches, eight to twelve times before lowering.

For Good Form and Safety:
- Push evenly off the ball of your foot so that your leg travels straight up and down.
- Apply downward hand pressure *behind* your knees rather than directly on top of them.

134

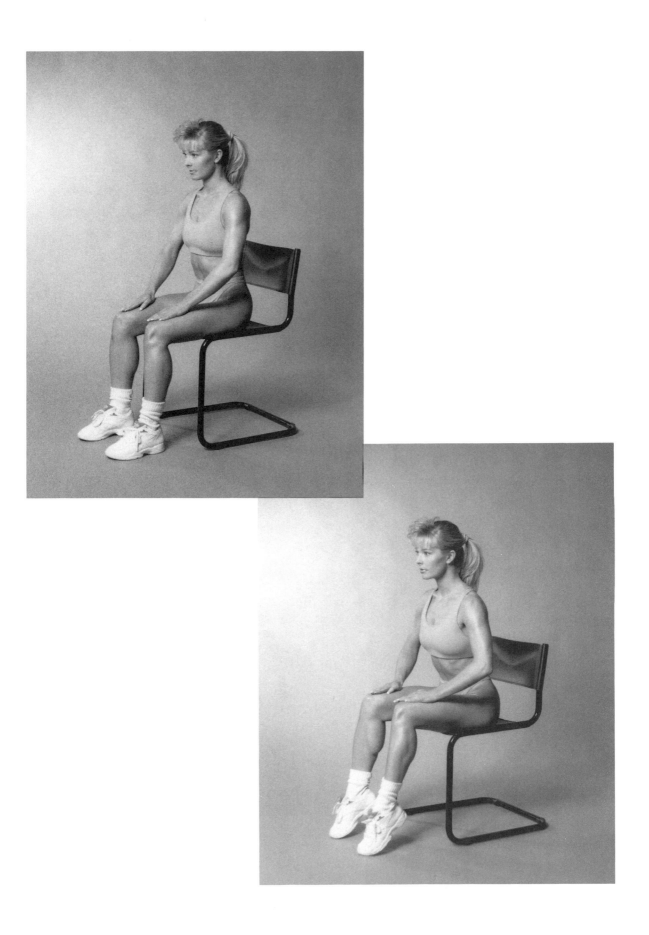

Leg Routines

Here are three leg routines you can try. Figure out how much time you want to spend target toning your legs (ten, fifteen, or twenty minutes), then adapt that routine to your level. Once you've tried our routines for a while, feel free to mix and match the exercises in this chapter to make up your own routines.

Equipment you'll need: A wall, step, exercise band or tube, mat, and a chair to use for sitting and as a stable object.

Optional for variations: One or two sets of risers, one or more sets of dumbbells.

How Many Reps Should I Do?

Do eight to fifteen repetitions each set. When you can do fifteen repetitions easily and with good form, move on to a more difficult variation of that exercise the next time you work out. If you find it difficult to do at least eight repetitions while maintaining good form, try an easier version of the exercise.

The only exception to this is the wall sit. When you can do three repetitions of fifteen seconds each, increase your sitting time by five seconds.

How Much Weight Should I Use?

When using resistance (dumbbell, ankle weight, or exercise band), choose a weight that will allow you to complete eight to fifteen repetitions with proper form. Increase the weight when you can do fifteen reps easily and with good form; if you can't get through at least eight reps, decrease the weight.

Beginners, try the exercises in this chapter without dumbbells or ankle weights; if you need to, you can add a three- to five-pound dumbbell or a one- to two-pound ankle weight. Always use the exercise band when it's called for in the basic description of an exercise. Intermediates, five- to ten-pound dumbbells and two- to three-pound ankle weights should provide enough resistance for the exercises in this chapter. Advanced, start with ten- to twelve-pound dumbbells and three- to five-pound ankle weights. These suggestions are guidelines only. Use a weight that feels challenging but that you can still handle comfortably. And keep in mind that you may not always use the same amount of resistance for every exercise.

How Much Should I Rest Between Sets?

Rest from thirty to ninety seconds between each exercise set. This will allow your muscles enough time to recover so they are strong enough to work their hardest when you do the next set but will not be so long that you lose the intensity and focus of your workout. You'll find that as you become stronger, you won't need as much rest between sets.

How Often Should I Target Tone My Legs?

For best results, target tone your legs three times a week with at least one day of rest in between each workout session.

Leg Isolation Routines

10-Minute Routine

(Beginner)

ORDER	EXERCISE	RESISTANCE/VARIATION	SETS
1	Wall Sit	Hold 15 seconds	1
2	One Leg Quad Pulse	None	1
3	Standing Leg Extension with Band	Exercise band	1
4	Step and Curl	None	2
5	Kneeling Four-Count Leg Curl with Band	Exercise band	1
6	Standing Calf Raise off Step	None	1

(INTERMEDIATE)

ORDER	EXERCISE	RESISTANCE/VARIATION	SETS
1	Wall Sit	Hold 15 seconds	1
2	One Leg Quad Pulse	Dumbbell	1
3	Standing Leg Extension with Band	Exercise band	1
4	Step and Curl	None	2
5	Kneeling Four-Count Leg Curl with Band	Exercise band	1
6	Standing Calf Raise off Step	8–12 pulses at top	1

(ADVANCED)

ORDER	EXERCISE	RESISTANCE/VARIATION	SETS
1	Wall Sit	Wall slide (pg. 118)	1
2	One Leg Quad Pulse	Dumbbell	1
3	Bump Squat	None	1
4	Step and Curl	None	2
5	Kneeling Four-Count Leg Curl with Band	Exercise band	1
6	Standing Calf Raise off Step	8–12 pulses at top	1

HOT BODY TIP

Are there any advantages to working out at a particular time of day? Research has shown that early birds tend to be more dedicated exercisers but are also more injury prone. Those who exercise later must navigate through a full day's worth of excuses and scheduling snafus but are less likely to get injured.

15-MINUTE ROUTINE

(BEGINNER)

ORDER	EXERCISE	RESISTANCE/VARIATION	SETS
1	Wall Sit	Hold for 15 seconds	1
2	One Leg Quad Pulse	None	2
3	Standing Leg Extension with Band	Exercise band	1
4	Bump Squat	None	1
5	Step and Curl	None	1
6	Kneeling Four-Count Leg Curl	Exercise band	1
7	Standing Leg Curl with Band	Exercise band	1
8	Standing Calf Raise off Step	None	1

(INTERMEDIATE)

ORDER	EXERCISE	RESISTANCE/VARIATION	SETS
1	Wall Sit	Hold for 15 seconds	1
2	One Leg Quad Pulse	Dumbbell	2
3	Standing Leg Extension with Band	Exercise band; pulse 12 times at top	1
4	Bump Squat	None	1
5	Step and Curl	None	1
6	Kneeling Four-Count Leg Curl	Exercise band	1
7	Standing Leg Curl with Band	Exercise band	1
8	Standing Calf Raise off Step	Dumbbell	1

(ADVANCED)

ORDER	EXERCISE	RESISTANCE/VARIATION	SETS
1	Wall Sit	Wall slide (pg. 118)	1
2	One Leg Quad Pulse	Dumbbell	2
3	Standing Leg Extension with Band	Exercise band; pulse 12 times at top	1
4	Bump Squat	Stand on tiptoe	1
5	Step and Curl	Dumbbells	1
6	Kneeling Four-Count Leg Curl	Exercise band	1
7	Standing Leg Curl with Band	Exercise band; pulse 12 times at top	1
8	Standing Calf Raise off Step	Dumbbell	1

20-MINUTE ROUTINE

(BEGINNER)

ORDER	EXERCISE	RESISTANCE/VARIATION	SETS
1	One Leg Quad Pulse	None	2
2	Standing Leg Extension with Band	None	1
3	Bump Squat	None	2
4	Step and Curl	None	2
5	Kneeling Four-Count Leg Curl	Exercise band	1
6	Standing Leg Curl with Band	Exercise band	1
7	Standing Calf Raise off Step	None	1
8	Seated Calf Raise	With step	1

(Intermediate)

ORDER	EXERCISE	RESISTANCE/VARIATION	SETS
1	One Leg Quad Pulse	Dumbbell	2
2	Standing Leg Extension with Band	Exercise band; pulse 12 times at top	1
3	Bump Squat	None	2
4	Step and Curl	Dumbbells	2
5	Kneeling Four-Count Leg Curl	Exercise band	1
6	Standing Leg Curl with Band	Exercise band; pulse at top	1
7	Standing Calf Raise off Step	Dumbbell	1
8	Seated Calf Raise	None	1

(Advanced)

ORDER	EXERCISE	RESISTANCE/VARIATION	SETS
1	One Leg Quad Pulse	Dumbbell; lower to squat position	2
2	Standing Leg Extension with Band	Exercise band; pulse 12 times at top	1
3	Bump Squat	Stand on tiptoe	2
4	Step and Curl	Dumbbells	2
5	Kneeling Four-Count Leg Curl	Exercise band; pulse at top	1
6	Standing Leg Curl with Band	Exercise band; pulse at top	1
7	Standing Calf Raise off Step	Dumbbell; one leg at a time	1
8	Seated Calf Raise	With step	1

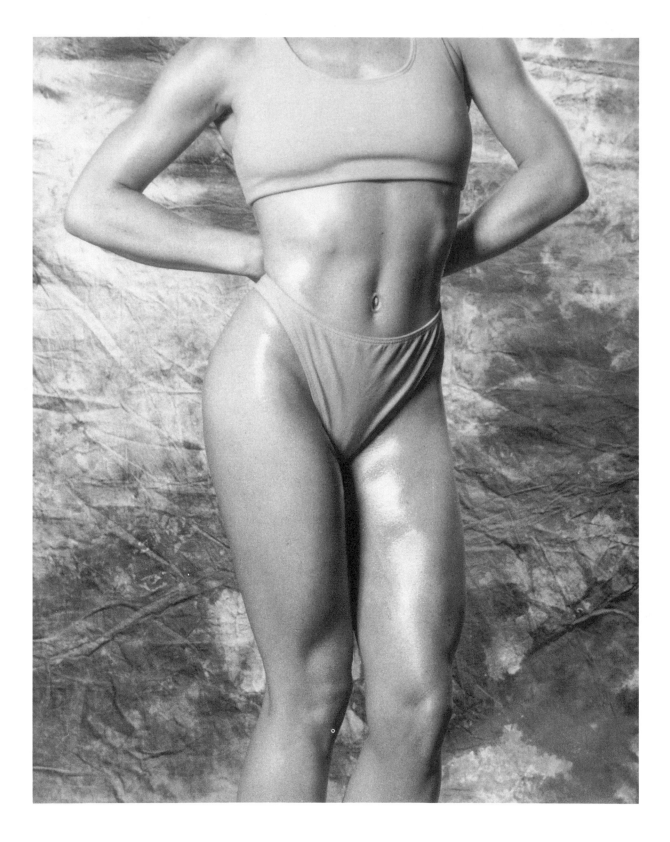

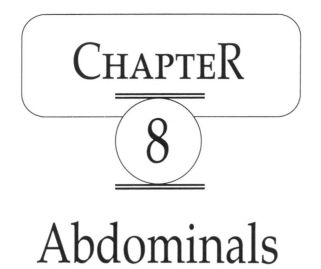

CHAPTER 8

Abdominals

For many of us, there's no fitness goal more sought after than a flat stomach. Fortunately, since the abdominals are easy to zero in on, they're a good candidate for target toning. The Buns of Steel abdominal routine will firm up your abs and whittle your middle. Your entire midsection will be tighter, sleeker, and slimmer. So get ready to throw away your baggy sweaters! You'll love what the exercises in this chapter will do for the appearance of your midriff.

These moves *will* help you firm your middle muscles. However, body fat is the ultimate difference between having a stomach that's strong but a bit rounded and one that's sleek and defined. Getting plenty of aerobic exercise and eating a healthy, low-fat diet will maximize your results.

These moves can do a lot more for you than just sculpting a set of killer abs. Want to pick up your posture? Strengthening your abdominals will help you stand up straighter. Are you striving to excel in a sport or fitness activity? A solid center will make you a better athlete by giving you more power from the middle. Are you pregnant? Stronger abs will make your delivery easier, and you'll bounce back into shape faster after your baby is born. Strengthening your abdominals will also help you reduce or avoid lower back pain. That's a real bonus when you consider that 80 percent of adult Americans experience back pain at some point in their lives.

Everyone can improve the appearance and strength of their abdominal area by doing the exercises in this chapter. The key is quality, not quantity. Forget the stories you've heard about celebrities who do three agonizing hours of sit-ups a day. Abdominals should be trained the same way as any other muscle group. By doing three or four well-focused target toning sessions a week, you'll see noticeable results in about six weeks.

Bottom line: If you do your abdominal work consistently, we guarantee you'll see a change. There's a good chance you'll feel these exercises working the very first time you try them. You'll probably notice that you're stronger and standing a little taller in just a couple of workouts.

The Abdominal Muscles

The *rectus abdominus* is a long, continuous wall of muscle that runs from your rib cage to your pubic bone. Anytime you bend at the middle you're using this muscle. Technically speaking, there are no "upper" and "lower" abs. Though you can originate a movement at either end, any exercise you do for the rectus works the entire muscle. "Reverse curl"–type movement places a bit more emphasis on the lower rectus muscle fibers; any movement that involves a "crunching" type movement places a bit more emphasis on the upper rectus muscle fibers.

Whenever you bend or twist to the side you bring the *internal* and *external obliques* into play. These are your true "waist" muscles. The *transversus abdominus* is located underneath the rectus. Although it doesn't initiate any body movements such as abdominal crunching or curling, they contract strongly when you pull your abdominals inward and then exhale—that's one reason why it's so important to maintain good form and breathe properly when doing abdominal exercises.

This chapter gives you nine separate abdominal exercises, and arranges them into routines specialized for *your* fitness level.

ABDOMINAL EXERCISES

1. Abdominal Grounding
2. Basic Crunch
3. Crossover Crunch
4. Total Crunch
5. Crunch and Pulse
6. Circular Crunch
7. Reverse Curl
8. Incline Reverse Curl
9. Waist Bend with Band

HOT BODY TIP

Before helping yourself to seconds, wait twenty minutes. While waiting, sip a glass of water, seltzer, or tea. Chances are your brain will signal your stomach that you're full and your urge to indulge will subside. If you're prone to wolfing down a single large portion, take your usual amount, place half of it on a separate plate, and resolve to wait at least twenty minutes before eating the second half. Or create the illusion of plenty by filling up a smaller plate.

HOT BODY TIP

When you grab a fast-food lunch at the mall, keep it simple. Stick to the single or junior versions rather than big-name specialty sandwiches. Hold the sauce, cheese, bacon, dressing, and anything that's fried in fat or oil. Plain cheese pizza, at 180 calories per slice, tops the list of safe, quick-grab selections. A plain hamburger at 250 calories or a basic chicken taco at 186 calories are also good choices. Tread lightly around salad bars: you can pile on more than 1,000 extra calories by using just a quarter cup of regular dressing, two ounces of cheese, a handful of nuts, and a few olives.

Exercise 1: ABDOMINAL GROUNDING

TARGET AREAS
This move teaches the proper method for using your abs and placing your back in a safe position for all floor exercises. Additionally, it target tones your abdominals.

The Setup: Lie on your back on your mat with your knees bent. Place your feet hip width apart and flat on the floor. Clasp your hands together and extend your arms straight along the floor above your head.

The Move:
• Round your lower back into the floor by pulling your abdominal muscles in toward your spine and tilting your pelvis upward.
• Lift your arms up until they are directly over your shoulders and, keeping your knee bent at a 90-degree angle and your foot flexed, raise your right leg until your knee is directly over your hip.
• Keep your lower back in firm contact with the floor as you slowly lower your arms and leg to the starting position.
• Switch legs and do an equal number of repetitions.

Mind/Body Focus: Think of your back as being anchored to the floor; don't allow the anchor to be lifted. This exercise will give you a sense of how your body should be positioned during any back-lying exercise. You'll feel tension along the entire length of your abdominal wall as you return to the start, especially if you move slowly and precisely.

For Good Form and Safety:
• Don't allow your neck or shoulders to come off the floor, and don't press your weight into the heel of your nonworking leg, as this may cause you to arch your lower back. You'll find it most difficult to maintain proper form the closer your leg moves toward the floor.
• Breathe naturally during this exercise.

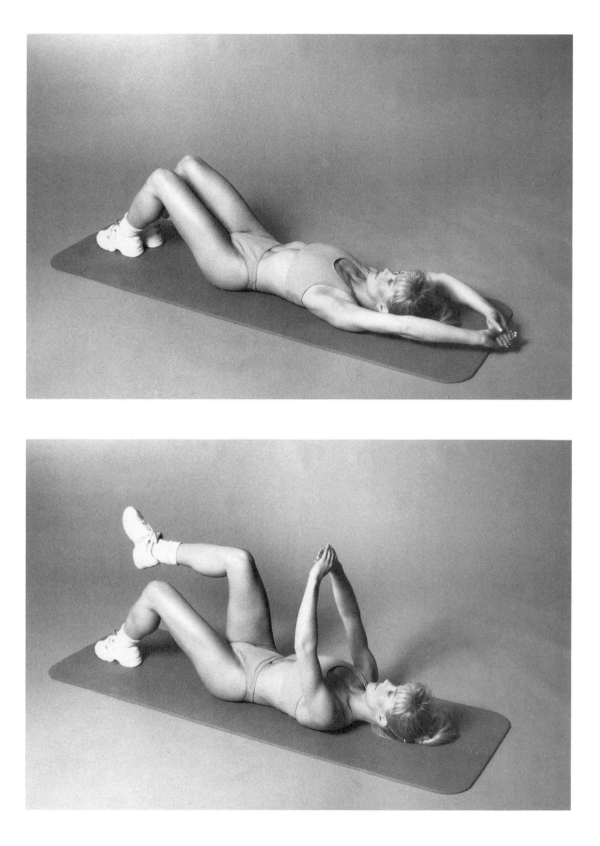

Exercise 2: BASIC CRUNCH

TARGET AREAS
This move is initiated in the upper muscle fibers of the abdominal wall and works the entire length of the muscle.

The Setup: Lie on your back with your knees bent and your feet hip width apart and flat on the floor. Place your hands behind your head so that your thumbs are behind your ears.

Don't lace your fingers together. Hold your elbows out wide enough so you can just see them out of the corners of your eyes and tilt your head back slightly. Round your lower back into the floor by gently pulling your abdominals in toward your spine and tilting your pelvis gently upward.

The Move:
- Exhale. Curl your spine up and forward so that your head, neck, and shoulder blades lift off the floor. There's no need to lift higher.
- Hold for a moment at the top of the movement, then inhale and lower slowly till just before the start.
- Move immediately into the next repetition.

Mind/Body Focus: During the upward phase, imagine someone is about to drop a weight onto your stomach from a height—you'll need to tense your abs in order to brace yourself for the impact. You'll feel tension just below your rib cage as you curl upward; this tension will spread through the entire abdominal area as you near completion of the set.

Variations:
- If this move is too difficult, fold your arms across your chest and tuck your chin so that it rests on your hands.
- To increase resistance, you can hold one arm straight out in back of you or, with both hands, hold a light dumbbell on top of your head.
- For more of a challenge, hold at the top of the movement for a slow count of five or pulse eight to twelve times, one to two inches at the top of the movement.

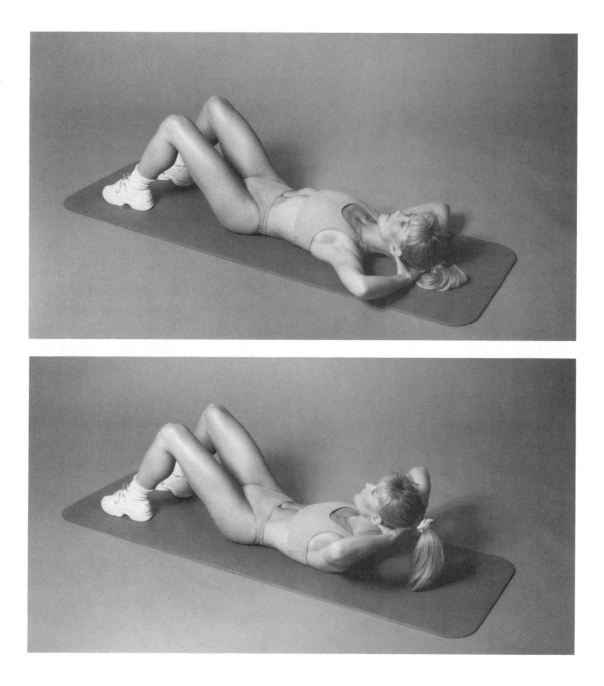

For Good Form and Safety:

- Keep your lower back firmly grounded, and don't lift upward by pulling on your neck with your hands. If you feel this move in your neck, you're either doing it incorrectly or need to practice an easier version till you become stronger.
- It's important to align your spine for this exercise, including your neck. To prevent your neck from hyperextending, leave a fist's worth of space between your chin and chest.

Exercise 3: CROSSOVER CRUNCH

TARGET AREAS
The abdominals and waist.

The Setup: Lie on your back with your right knee bent and your left ankle crossed over your right knee. Place your hands behind your head so that your thumbs are behind your ears. *Don't lace your fingers together.* Hold your elbows out wide and tilt your head back slightly. Round your lower back into the floor by gently pulling your abdominals in toward your spine and tilting your pelvis gently upward.

The Move:
- Exhale. Curl your head, neck, and shoulder blades up off the floor, and as you curl upward, move your right elbow toward your left knee (you don't have to touch it).
- Inhale and lower slowly till you are just above the start. Immediately begin the next rep.
- Switch legs and do the same number of reps to the other side.

Mind/Body Focus: As you curl upward and sideways, pretend you are trying to bump something out of the way with your shoulder. You'll feel this in your abdominals in the upward phase and your waist on the side you're crossing toward.

Variations:
- If you find this move too difficult, keep both feet flat on the floor.
- To make this exercise more advanced, start with both your knees bent, and lift your bent knees off the floor and cross one ankle over the other.
- You can add more "resistance" to this exercise by reaching with your arm extended rather than using your elbow.

For Good Form and Safety:
- Twist from the abdominals rather than simply moving your elbow in the direction of your knee.
- Take care that the entire movement is done with your abs and waist muscles, not by pulling upward on your neck with your hands.

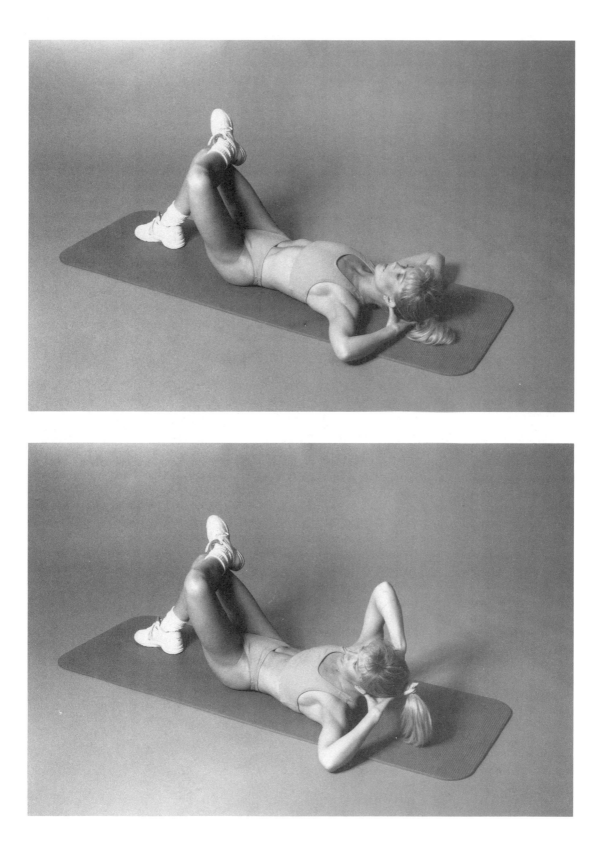

Exercise 4: TOTAL CRUNCH

TARGET AREAS
Movement originates from both the upper and lower fibers of the abdominal muscles. Works the entire abdominal wall.

The Setup: Lie on your back with your knees bent. Place your hands behind your head so that your thumbs are behind your ears. *Don't lace your fingers together.* Hold your elbows out wide, tilt your head back slightly, and round your lower back into the floor by gently pulling your abdominals in toward your spine. Lift your legs so that your thighs are directly over your hips. At the topmost position your knees should be bent at a 90-degree angle.

The Move:
- Exhale. Slowly curl your head, neck, and shoulder blades upward and forward off the floor. At the same time, curl upward from the hips so that your knees travel back toward your elbows. At the top of the movement your knees and elbows will be separated by a few inches.
- Hold for a moment, inhale, and lower slowly till you are just above the start.
- Move immediately into the next repetition.

Mind/Body Focus: This move should be done slowly so it isn't powered by momentum. As you crunch, imagine you're an armadillo trying to curl itself into a protective ball. You'll feel your abdominal muscles working during the upward phase of this movement.

Variations:
- To make this exercise easier, cross one ankle over the opposite knee.
- To isolate upper and lower muscle fibers, alternate upper and lower body movements.
- For more of a challenge, hold at the top for a slow five count or pulse eight to twelve times, one to two inches at the top of the movement.

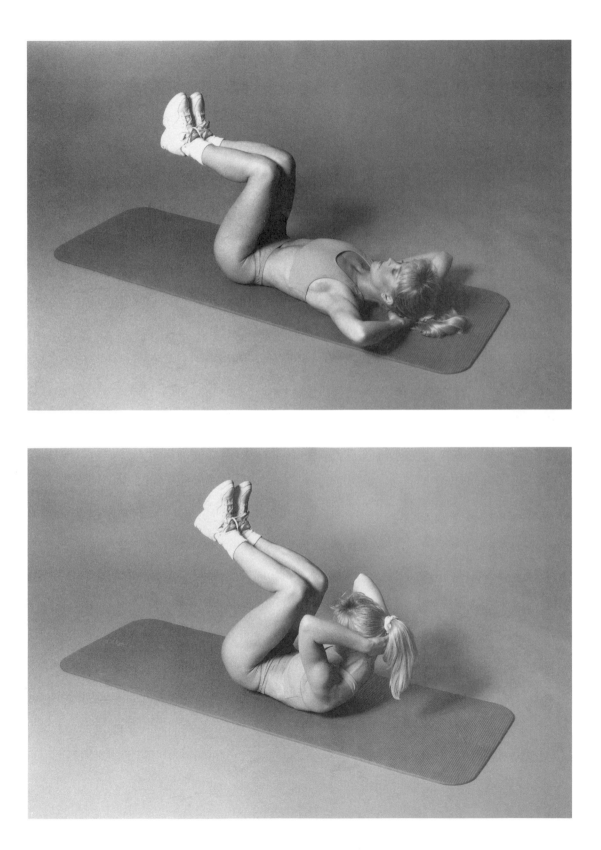

Exercise 5: CRUNCH AND PULSE

TARGET AREAS
Works the entire abdominal wall.

The Setup: Lie on your back with your legs extended straight up over your hips and your knees slightly bent. Raise your arms straight up over your chest toward your toes. Tuck your chin under so that there's a fist's worth of space between your chin and chest. Round your lower back into the floor by gently pulling your abdominals in toward your spine.

The Move:
• Exhale. Curl your upper body upward until your shoulder blades clear the floor and slide your arms up the front of your legs a few inches until your fingertips reach the tops of your ankles (or as far as you can). Hold in this position for a moment until you feel a strong contraction in your abs.
• Inhale and lower to the start.

Mind/Body Focus: Imagine you're trying to brush something off your legs that's just out of reach. Done correctly, it will create a feeling of continuous tension in your abdominal muscles as you do these small upward and downward movements.

Variations:
• If you need to support your head and neck, hold one hand behind your head and reach up with the other.
• Bring your sides or "obliques" into play by reaching across to one side then the other as you pulse.

For Good Form and Safety:
• Don't do this movement in a quick or jerky manner, or you may feel it in your lower back or neck.
• If your flexibility doesn't allow you to straighten your legs, it's okay to bend your knees as much as you need.

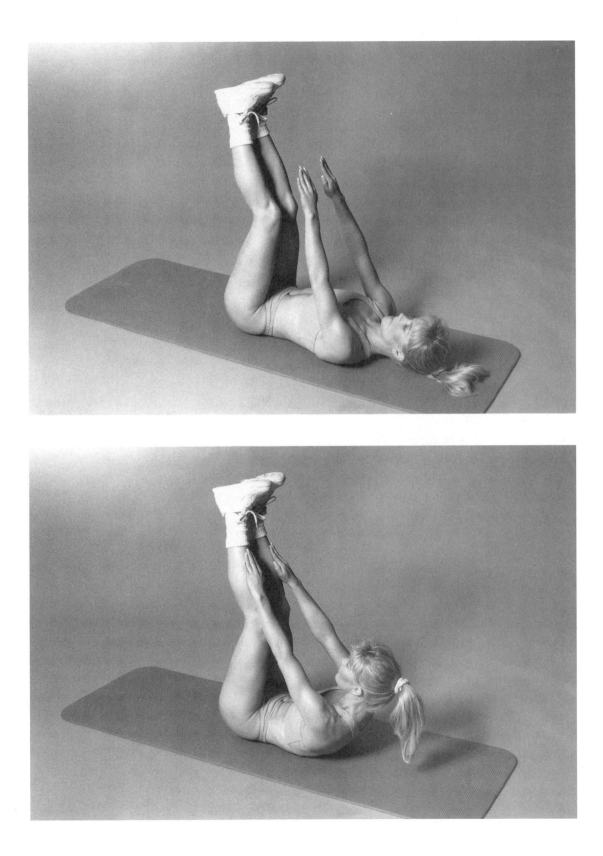

Exercise 6: CIRCULAR CRUNCH

TARGET AREAS
This very intense move thoroughly works your abdominals and waist.

The Setup: Lie on your back with your knees bent and your feet hip width apart and flat on the floor. Place your hands behind your head so that your thumbs are behind your ears. *Don't lace your fingers together.* Hold your elbows out wide, tilt your head back slightly, and round your lower back into the floor by gently pulling your abdominals in toward your spine.

The Move:
- Lift your head, neck, and shoulder blades off the floor and hold at the top of the movement.
- Make a small clockwise circle with your waist: bend a small distance to the left, curl a small distance upward, move through center to bend a small distance to the right, and then lower a small distance downward to the start.
- This is one repetition.
- Exhale and inhale on alternate repetitions.
- Do an equal number of reps in a counterclockwise direction.

Mind/Body Focus: Done correctly this movement is very subtle, very fluid—similar to a belly dancer's. Each small, precise circle should trace the orbit of the previous circle. During this exercise you'll feel a continuous contraction in the muscles of your abdominals and waist.

For Good Form and Safety:
- This move is initiated with your abdominal and oblique muscles only.
- Keeping your circles small and doing them slowly will help you avoid pulling upward on your neck with your hands.

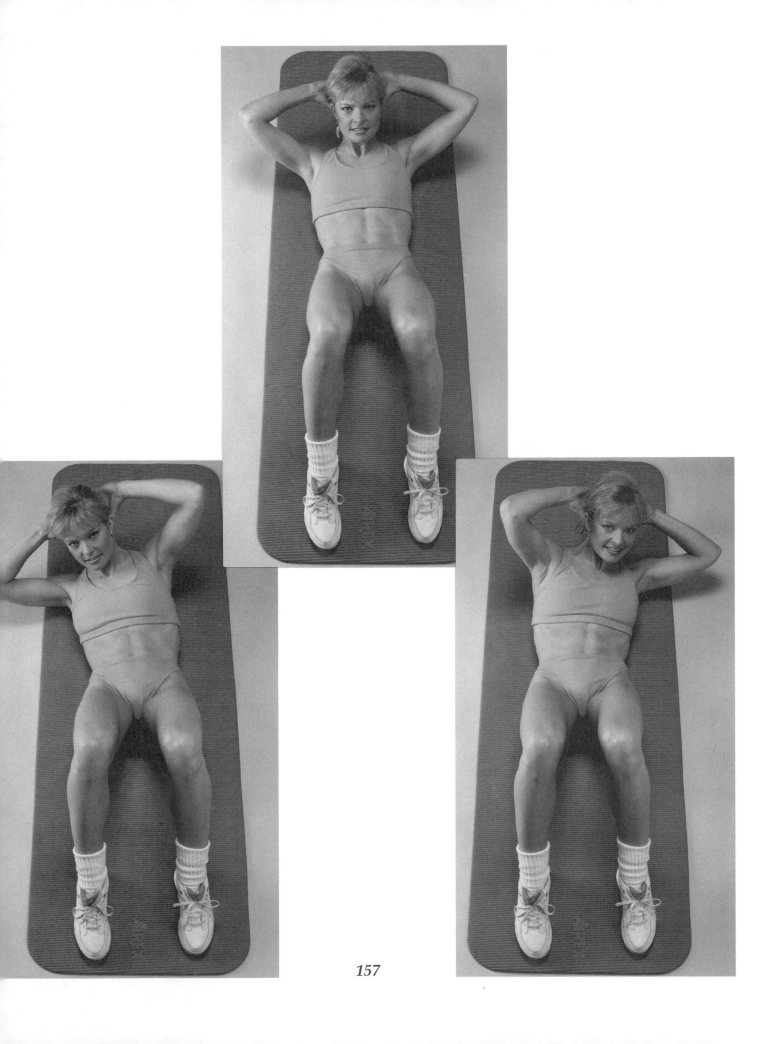

157

Exercise 7: REVERSE CURL

TARGET AREAS

Movement originates from the lower part of the abs and works the entire abdominal wall.

The Setup: Lie on your back with your knees bent. Lift your legs so that your thighs are directly over your hips and your calves are parallel to the floor. Rest your arms at your sides with your palms facing downward. Round your lower back into the floor by gently pulling your abdominals in toward your spine.

The Move:

- Exhale. Lift your tailbone directly upward so that your buttocks raise about an inch off the floor.
- In this lifted position, roll your hips a few inches back so that your knees travel toward your chest.
- Inhale and slowly lower to the start.

Mind/Body Focus: Although we've broken up this move into two distinctive phases to describe it—a lift upward and a roll backward—it should be done in one smooth, fluid movement, like a rocking chair being rocked by a soft breeze. Done correctly, it will create a feeling of tension just below your belly button as you lift and rock; this tension will spread through your entire abdominal wall as you reach the end of the set.

Variations:

- To add resistance, use an exercise tube. One with handles works best. Wrap the tubing around both ankles to form a loop around each. Hold an end or handle firmly in each hand and pull them down to hold them close to your buttocks. Every time you rock backward, the band should become taut.

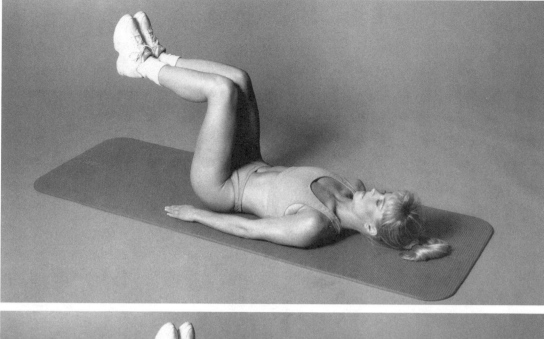

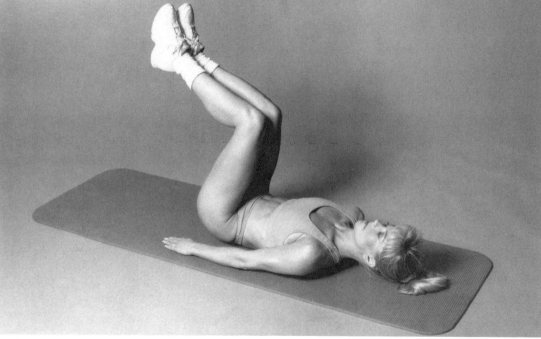

For Good Form and Safety:

- Don't allow your lower back to arch off the floor as you lower. You should *not* feel your lower back working.
- Do this movement slowly to take all the momentum out of it. There's no need to exaggerate it, either: lifting your buttocks an inch upward and rolling your hips slightly backward will be more effective than going through a larger range of motion.

Exercise 8: INCLINE REVERSE CURL

TARGET AREAS
Movement originates from the lower part of your abs and works the entire abdominal wall.

The Setup: Place two risers securely underneath one end of your step. (You can also use an incline bench.) Lie on the step on your back so that your head is at the higher end and your spine, including your neck, is perfectly aligned. Grasp the underside of the top end of the step with one hand on either side of your head. Lift your feet off the step, and bend your legs so that the tops of your knees are positioned just behind your hips and your calves are parallel to the floor.

The Move:
• Lift your tailbone upward, raising your buttocks one inch off the step.
• As you reach this up position, roll your hips a few inches back so that your knees travel toward your chest.
• Inhale and lower slowly to the start.

Mind/Body Focus: Doing this exercise with your head at the higher end of the step forces you to lift against gravity. You should feel tension just below your belly button as you lift and roll back; this tension will spread through your entire abdominal muscle as you reach the end of the set.

Variations:
• If you find this exercise too difficult, remove one riser from both ends so that you have one at the higher end and none at the lower. Or, you can lie in the opposite direction, with your head at the lower part of the step.
• Build a higher incline by adding an additional riser underneath the inclined end of the step to make this more challenging.

For Good Form and Safety:
• You should *not* feel your lower back working, nor should you force the movement by pulling with your arms.

160

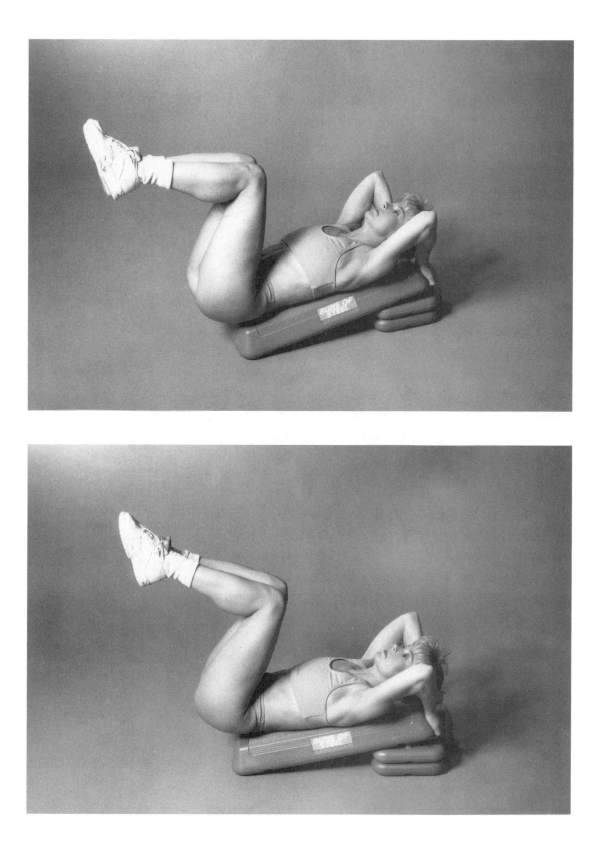

Exercise 9: WAIST BEND WITH BAND

TARGET AREAS
Target tones the waist (internal and external obliques).

The Setup: Stand with your feet a bit more than hip width apart on the center of an exercise tube or band. With your arms at your sides, hold on to a handle or end with each hand; bend your elbows slightly and face your palms inward. Stand up tall and maintain a natural curve in your spine.

The Move:
- Exhale, bend your waist to the left, and tilt your left hip about one-half inch upward.
- Inhale. Return to the start.
- In the same manner, bend to the right.
- Alternate sides, and do an equal number of repetitions to each side.

Mind/Body Focus: You should feel a contraction on the outside and center of your waist on the side you are bending toward. You'll feel a stretch on the opposite side.

Variations:
- If you find this exercise too difficult, do it without the band.
- To increase the resistance, shorten the band or use a stronger band.

For Good Form and Safety:
- As you bend to the side, keep your arms still and your shoulders down and relaxed—and don't arch your back.
- Keep the movement small and precise for maximum effectiveness.
- To prevent the band from sliding out from under your feet, start by standing on the center of the band and then moving one foot out to the side so that your feet are hip width apart and there is about ten inches of band between both feet.

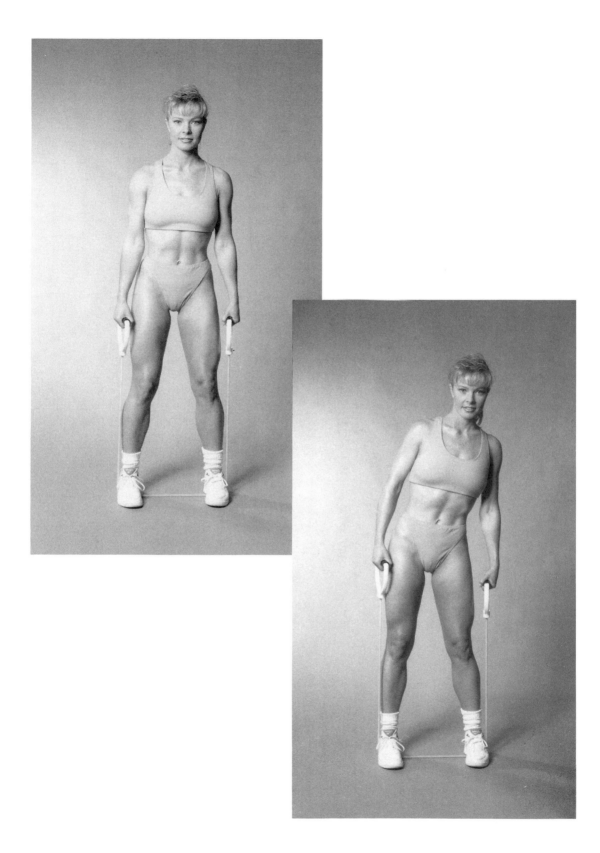

Abdominal Routines

Here are three abdominal routines you can try. Figure out how much time you want to spend target toning your abs (ten, fifteen, or twenty minutes), then adapt that routine to your level. Once you've tried our routines for a while and you get a sense of what works for you, by all means mix and match our exercises to put together your own routines.

Equipment you'll need: A mat, a step with one or two sets of risers, and an exercise band or tube.

Optional for variations: One or more sets of dumbbells.

How Many Reps Should I Do?

Do eight to fifteen repetitions each set, just as you would when working any other muscle group. When you can do fifteen repetitions easily and with good form, move on to a more difficult variation of that exercise the next time you work out. If you find it difficult to do at least eight repetitions while maintaining good form, try an easier version of the exercise. This is much more effective than doing more than fifty repetitions per set as you may have done with other body-shaping programs.

How Much Weight Should I Use?

For most abdominal exercises, you'll find that the weight of your own body will provide plenty of resistance. Only one variation of the basic crunch and one variation of the reverse curl call for any additional resistance, a dumbbell and exercise band, respectively.

How Much Should I Rest Between Sets?

Rest from thirty to ninety seconds between each exercise set. This will allow your muscles enough time to recover so they are strong enough to work their hardest when you do the next set but will not be so long that you lose the intensity and focus of your workout. You'll find that as you become stronger, you won't need as much rest between sets.

How Often Should I Target Tone My Abs?

For best results, target tone your abs three to four times a week with at least one day of rest in between each workout session.

Abdominal Isolation Routine

10-MINUTE ROUTINE

(BEGINNER)

ORDER	EXERCISE	RESISTANCE/VARIATION	SETS
1	Abdominal Grounding	None	1
2	Basic Crunch	None	2
3	Crossover Crunch	None	1
4	Reverse Curl	None	2
5	Waist Bend with Band	Exercise band	1

HOT BODY TIP

The time to drink is *before* you're thirsty. Drink plenty of fluids before, during, and after your workouts, especially on hot days. Water and sports drinks are your best choices. Soft drinks, caffeinated beverages, and fruit juices have been known to cause cramps.

(Intermediate)

ORDER	EXERCISE	RESISTANCE/VARIATION	SETS
1	Abdominal Grounding	None	1
2	Basic Crunch	Dumbbell	2
3	Crossover Crunch	Extend arm upward	1
4	Reverse Curl	Exercise band	2
5	Waist Bend with Band	Exercise band	1

(Advanced)

ORDER	EXERCISE	RESISTANCE/VARIATION	SETS
1	Abdominal Grounding	None	1
2	Total Crunch	Alternate upper and lower body	2
3	Crossover Crunch	Extend arm upward	1
4	Incline	None	2
5	Waist Bend with Band	Exercise band	1

HOT BODY TIP

Recent studies indicate that besides being loaded with empty calories (a hundred calories an ounce or more), alcohol may actually inhibit fat loss because your body may burn calories that come from alcohol before calories derived from food. No-cal sodas and fruit juices mixed with seltzer are ideal substitutes for toasting festive occasions. Or use one of the following strategies to limit your alcohol intake: set a cutoff time for yourself, say, 9:30 P.M., after which you will drink only nonalcoholic beverages; follow every alcoholic drink you have with a glass of water; or start out with a regular drink, and when it's half gone, add water or seltzer.

15-Minute Routine
(Beginner)

ORDER	EXERCISE	RESISTANCE/VARIATION	SETS
1	Abdominal Grounding	None	1
2	Basic Crunch	None	2
3	Crossover Crunch	None	2
4	Total Crunch	None	1
5	Circular Crunch	None	1
6	Reverse Curl	None	2

(Intermediate)

ORDER	EXERCISE	RESISTANCE/VARIATION	SETS
1	Abdominal Grounding	None	1
2	Basic Crunch	Hold 5 counts at top	2
3	Crossover Crunch	Extend one arm	2
4	Total Crunch	None	1
5	Circular Crunch	None	1
6	Reverse Curl	None	2

(Advanced)

ORDER	EXERCISE	RESISTANCE/VARIATION	SETS
1	Abdominal Grounding	None	1
2	Basic Crunch	Dumbbell; hold 5 counts at top	2
3	Crossover Crunch	Extend one arm	2
4	Total Crunch	Reach to side	1
5	Circular Crunch	None	1
6	Reverse Curl	Exercise band	2

20-Minute Routine
(Beginner)

ORDER	EXERCISE	RESISTANCE/VARIATION	SETS
1	Abdominal Grounding	None	1
2	Basic Crunch	None	2
3	Crossover Crunch	None	1
4	Total Crunch	None	1
5	Crunch and Pulse	None	1
6	Circular Crunch	None	1
7	Reverse Curl	None	1
8	Incline Reverse Curl	Lie with head at lower end of step	1
9	Waist Bend	Exercise band	2

(Intermediate)

ORDER	EXERCISE	RESISTANCE/VARIATION	SETS
1	Abdominal Grounding	None	1
2	Basic Crunch	Hold 5 counts at top	2
3	Crossover Crunch	Extend one arm	1
4	Total Crunch	None	1
5	Crunch and Pulse	None	1
6	Circular Crunch	None	1
7	Reverse Curl	None	1
8	Incline Reverse Curl	None	1
9	Waist Bend	Exercise band	2

(Advanced)

ORDER	EXERCISE	RESISTANCE/VARIATION	SETS
1	Abdominal Grounding	None	1
2	Basic Crunch	Hold 5 counts at top; add dumbbell	2
3	Crossover Crunch	Extend one arm	1
4	Total Crunch	Reach to side	1
5	Crunch and Pulse	None	1
6	Circular Crunch	None	1
7	Reverse Curl	Exercise band	1
8	Incline Reverse Curl	None	1
9	Waist Bend	Exercise band	2

HOT BODY TIP

It doesn't matter how fast you get there as long as you take the journey. One mile of walking burns only slightly fewer calories than running one mile. And it's less stressful on your body!

HOT BODY TIP

You can estimate your walking speed in steps per minute (SPM): 60 SPM = 2 miles per hour (MPH); 90 SPM = 3 MPH; and 120 SPM = 4 MPH.

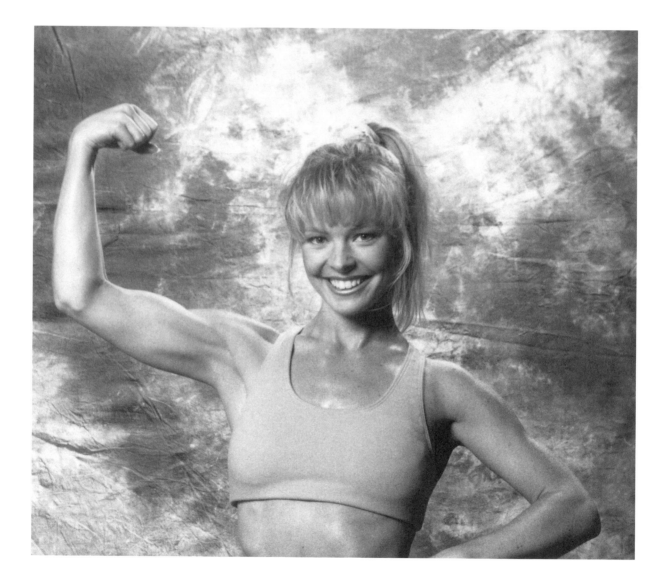

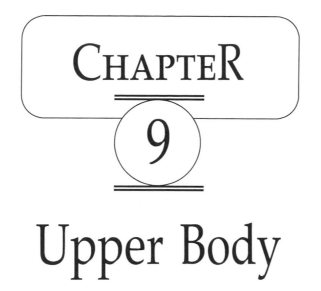

CHAPTER

9

Upper Body

You may not consider your upper body a problem area, but when your abs and lower body turn into steel, you'll want the proportion that comes from having the *total* picture. Fortunately your arms, chest, and upper back are places where you see results fast.

Doing the Buns of Steel upper body routine *will not* make you resemble a body builder. Only hours in the gym lifting heavy weights can do that—and then only one in a thousand women will be able to develop body-builder's proportions. Rather, your muscles will look tighter, firmer, and more sculpted.

Target toning your upper body will also help enhance your appearance from the waist down. A sculpted, beautifully muscled upper body will give you a well-balanced physique that will make your buns and legs look smaller. Your body will have symmetry and proportion, and you'll finally have that fit-from-head-to-toe body you've always wanted.

There's still another reason to pick up those weights and exercise bands: strength. Whether you're lifting heavy packages, opening a door against the wind, or carrying your own suitcases as you run to catch a plane, you rely on the strength of your upper body muscles. This extra strength will give you a feeling of independence and freedom because everything you do will be less of an effort.

The muscles in your upper body are all different shapes and sizes, so you may see them improve at different rates. Where you see improvements first will depend upon you as an individual. Some women see their chests firm up right away, while others develop a nice athletic V shape in their backs before they see any development anywhere else. Most women see an overall improvement in their appearance after four to six weeks of doing the Buns of Steel upper body target toning routines two to three times a week. You'll probably feel improvements in the form of extra strength much sooner. You'll be amazed when a weight that felt heavy during your first workout suddenly feels very light.

Upper Body Muscles

There are many muscles in your upper body. For the purposes of our discussion, we need touch upon only the basics.

The *latissimus dorsi*, which spans your entire upper back, is the largest muscle in your upper body. Every time you pull something toward you, you use this muscle. Your chest muscles, or the *pectorals*, are used in pushing things such as a lawn mower or a shopping cart. Your shoulder muscles, or *deltoids*, come into play just about any time you use your upper body, even when all you do is pick up or put down this book. Finally, the muscles in the front of your upper arms are called the *biceps* and the muscles in the back are the *triceps*. (The triceps in particular are a trouble spot for women, especially as they get older.) Any time you use your arms you can be sure these muscles are working.

This chapter details thirteen exercises targeted to your upper back, chest, shoulders, triceps, and biceps. Beginning, intermediate, and advanced routines allow you to fit a terrific targeted workout in whatever time you have available.

UPPER BODY EXERCISES

Upper Back

1. Pullover
2. Seated Row with Band
3. Lat Pulldown with Band

Chest

4. Push-up
5. Chest Fly
6. Crossover with Band

Shoulders

7. Shoulder Press
8. Lateral Raise
9. Upright Row with Band

Triceps

10. Kickback
11. Triceps Extension with Band

Biceps

12. Seated Biceps Curl
13. Standing Biceps Curl with Band

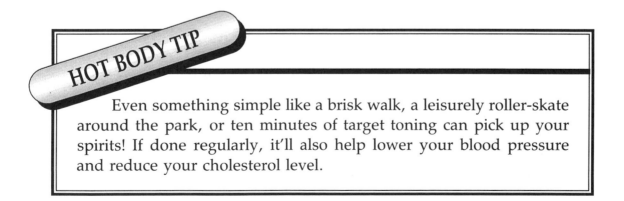

HOT BODY TIP

Even something simple like a brisk walk, a leisurely roller-skate around the park, or ten minutes of target toning can pick up your spirits! If done regularly, it'll also help lower your blood pressure and reduce your cholesterol level.

UPPER BACK

Exercise 1: PULLOVER

TARGET AREAS
A great overall upper body toner, this exercise emphasizes your upper back as well as your chest, shoulder, arms, and abdominals.

The Setup: For this exercise, use a step with two sets of risers underneath (four to six inches high). Lie on your step lengthwise with your knees bent, your feet flat on the floor, and your head resting on the end of the step. Grasp the underside of one end of a dumbbell in both of your hands with your palms facing upward and thumbs overlapping. Extend your arms slightly past your shoulders while keeping a slight bend in your elbows.

The Move:
- Inhale. Keeping the slight bend in your elbows, lower the dumbbell back behind your head in an arclike path, bending your arms until you feel a stretch in your rib cage and chest.
- Hold for a moment at the bottom of the movement for an additional stretch.
- Exhale and lift the weight back up to the start, retracing the arclike path.

Mind/Body Focus: Think of your arms as a link between the dumbbell and your upper back muscles—though your arms are moving, concentrate on powering the weight upward with your larger, stronger back muscles. If you do this correctly, you'll feel a stretch in your chest, shoulders, and rib cage as the weight moves downward and as you hold at the bottom; you'll feel the upward movement in your chest and the outer "wings" of your upper back.

Variations:
- If you find this move too difficult, do it lying on the floor to restrict the range of motion.

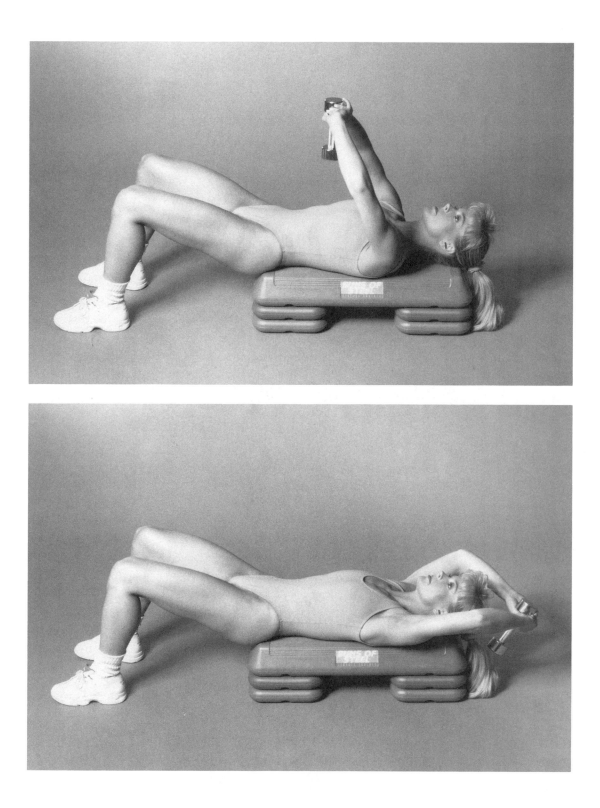

For Good Form and Posture:
- Don't allow your lower back to arch up off the step, especially as you near the bottom of the movement.

Exercise 2: SEATED ROW WITH BAND

TARGET AREAS
Target tones your upper back, shoulders, and the fronts of your arms.

The Setup: Sit on the floor with your legs hip width apart straight out in front of you with your knees slightly bent. Flex your feet. Wrap an exercise band or tube around the instep of both of your feet and, with your palms facing inward, grasp an end or handle in each hand. Bend your elbows so that your hands are brushing against your waist and the band is taut. Sit up tall and pull your abdominals inward.

The Move:
- Inhale. Straighten your arms and reach forward, *not by rounding your back*, but by bending forward from your hips. Lengthen out your body until your hands reach the top of your toes or come as far forward as your flexibility allows.
- Exhale and, leading with your elbows, bend your arms and pull the band back up to the start.

Mind/Body Focus: Imagine you're rowing a boat and the exercise band is your set of oars. In the lengthened-out position you'll feel a stretch in your arms, shoulders, lower back, and backs of your thighs. You'll feel your upper back and arm muscles working as you pull the band toward you.

Variations:
- To increase the resistance, shorten the band or use a stronger band.
- For a bigger challenge, do a one arm row. Cross one end or handle of the band over the other and grasp in one hand. Stretch that arm toward the opposite toe. As you come up twist slightly to the outside. Do an equal number of repetitions with both arms.
- To get an even longer stretch, loop the band around a stable object such as the leg of a bed or a pole so you can lengthen out past your toes.

For Good Form and Safety:
- Don't lower yourself by rounding your back—bend from the hips.
- If your lower back or thigh flexibility is limited, it's okay to bend your knees more than slightly.

176

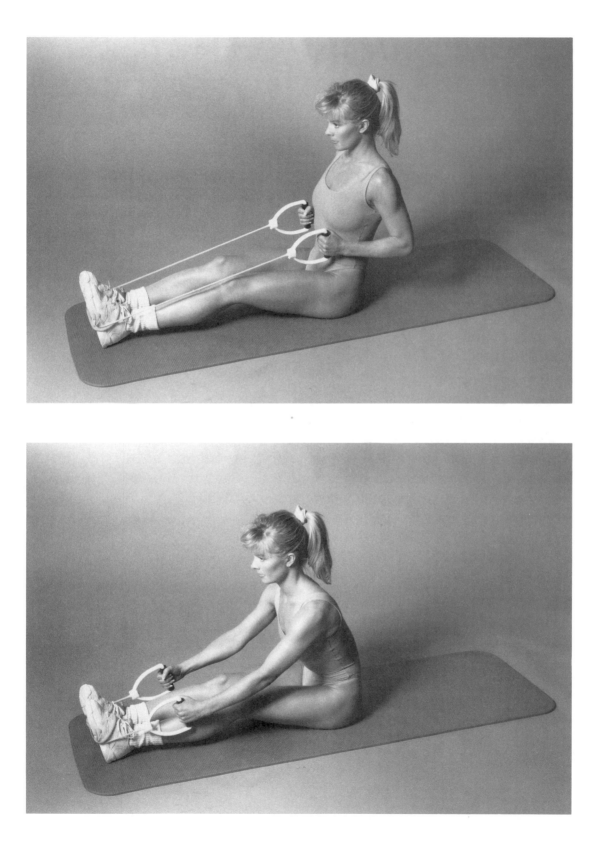

Exercise 3: LAT PULLDOWN WITH BAND

TARGET AREAS
Works your upper back, shoulders, and fronts of arms.

The Setup: Tie together the ends of an exercise band or tube; make sure the knot is secure. Stand with your feet hip width apart and hold this "band circle" in both hands. Raise your arms over your head with your palms facing downward and your elbows bent.

The Move:
- Keep your right arm as still as possible. Exhale. By bending your left elbow downward and out to the side, pull the band down to the left until your hand is almost level with the top of your shoulder. In the end position the band will be tight and your elbow will point down toward the floor.
- Inhale. Slowly raise your arm back to the start.
- Repeat the same movement with your other arm.
- Alternate arms. Do an equal number of repetitions with both arms.

Mind/Body Focus: Imagine you're shooting a bow and arrow straight up into the air. When you pull your arm down, you draw the bow tight; when you straighten your arm, you send the arrow flying. You'll feel tension in the outer "wings" of your upper back and the front of your arm as you pull downward.

Variations:
- Do all repetitions to one side, then the other.
- Pull both arms down at the same time.

For Good Form and Safety:
- Keep your wrists in line with the rest of your arms.
- To prevent your lower back from arching, stand tall by pulling your abdominals inward and maintaining a natural curve in your spine.

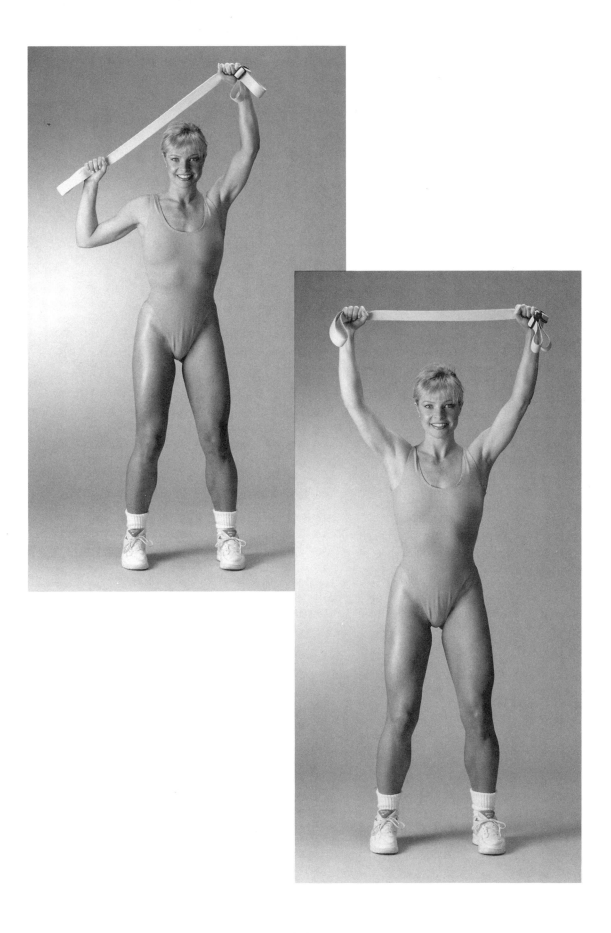

179

CHEST

Exercise 4: PUSH-UP

TARGET AREAS
Works the chest, shoulders, and backs of the upper arms. Since your abdominals help stabilize your body, they also get a good workout.

The Setup: Kneel down and position your hands and knees so that your knees are directly under your hips and your hands are slightly in front of your shoulders. Push yourself up by straightening your arms and extend your legs straight out behind you—you're supporting your weight on your toes and your hands. Pull your abdominals in, and keep your entire spine in a straight line.

The Move:
- Inhale. Lower your entire body toward the floor by bending your elbows down and out to the side.
- When you come as close as you can to touching your chest to the floor, exhale and raise up to the start.

Mind/Body Focus: Make sure you move your body as a single unit. In other words, don't lower your chest first, then your back, then your legs. You'll feel the muscles in your chest and the backs of your arms working as you push upward.

Variations:
- If this move is too difficult, do it from the kneeling position so there's a straight line from your head to your knees, and push off from your hands. Note: Don't be intimidated by the thought of doing a full push-up! Though most women are usually taught this "from the knees" version, with a little training you should be able to master the "legs out" position.
- If push-ups from the knees are still too tough, try a wall push-up: stand an arm's length away from a wall and place your hands on the wall slightly wider than shoulder width apart. Lower yourself toward the wall by bending your elbows. Keep your feet flat on the floor.

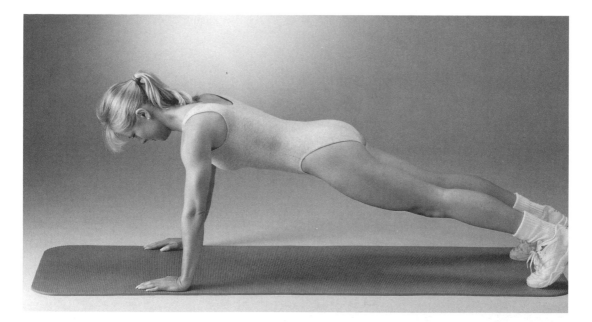

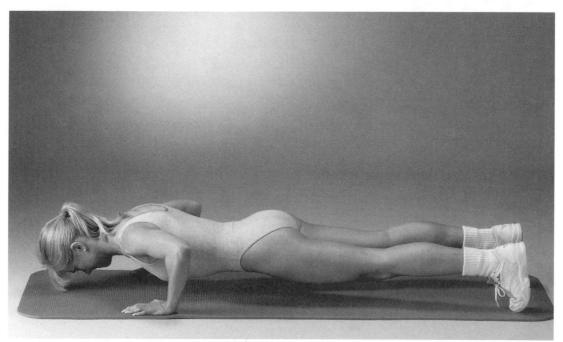

- To increase the difficulty, loop an exercise band or tube around your upper back and hold an end in each hand.

For Good Form and Safety:
- Be sure to keep your abdominals tight so they don't sag downward and cause your lower back to overarch.
- As you lower, bring your shoulder blades together rather than rounding your shoulders forward and dropping your neck.

Exercise 5: CHEST FLY

TARGET AREAS
Target tones the chest, shoulders, and backs of arms.

The Setup: Lie on your bench or step with two sets of risers underneath (four to six inches high), with your knees bent, feet flat on the floor, and your head resting on the step. Grasp a dumbbell in each hand and straighten your arms directly up over your shoulders so that your elbows are slightly bent, your palms are facing in, and the dumbbells are touching each other.

The Move:
- Inhale. Slowly lower your arms, bending your elbows a bit more and bringing your arms out to the side. In the most downward position your elbows will be bent about halfway and your hands will be a few inches above chest level.
- Hold for a moment at the bottom of the movement till you feel a stretch through your chest.
- Exhale and return to the start.

Mind/Body Focus: In the lowered position imagine you're hugging a big oak tree. You'll feel a stretch through your chest as you lower and hold the weights; you'll feel your chest muscles contract as you raise the weights back up to the start.

Variations:
- To emphasize the upper part of your chest muscles (from your shoulders to the top of your bra line), incline your weight bench about 45 degrees or place three risers under one end of your step and no risers underneath the other end. Lie with your head at the higher end and do the exercise exactly as you did on the flat surface.
- To emphasize the lower part of your chest muscles (from the midline of your bra to the band), lie with your head at the lower end.
- If you find this exercise too difficult, do it lying on the floor to restrict the distance the weights travel.

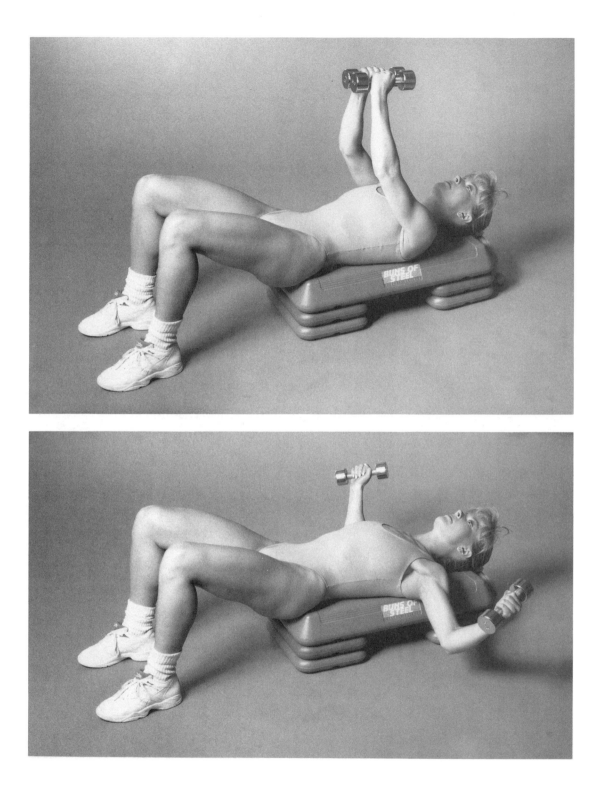

For Good Form and Safety:
• Pull your abdominals in toward your spine so that you don't allow your back to arch off the step, especially as you lower the weights.
• Keep your wrists in line with your forearms at all times.

Exercise 6: CROSSOVER WITH BAND

TARGET AREAS
Target tones your chest, shoulders, and backs of the arms.

The Setup: Run an exercise band or tube underneath your step. Lie on the step with your knees bent, your feet flat on the floor, your head resting on the step, and your elbows bent so that they point toward the floor and your hands are about three inches above chest level. Hold a handle or end of the band in each hand so that your palms are facing in and the band runs behind your elbows.

The Move:
• Exhale. Straighten your arms upward directly over your shoulders while maintaining a slight bend in your elbows. The band should get progressively tighter as you go.
• At the top of the movement, cross one wrist directly over the other.
• Inhale and lower slowly to the start.
• Alternate which wrist crosses in front until you have completed *all reps*.

Mind/Body Focus: This time you're hugging that giant oak tree at the *top* of the movement. You're doing this right if you feel tension in the muscles of your chest and the backs of your arms as you move upward. The tension in your chest will increase as you cross one wrist over the other.

Variations:
• If you find this move too difficult, do a bench press: eliminate the wrist cross and simply press straight upward directly over your chest.
• To emphasize the upper fibers of your chest (from the bottom of your neck to the center of your bra line), incline your weight bench or place three risers under one end of your step and no risers underneath the other end. Lie with your head at the higher end and do the exercise exactly as you did on the flat surface.
• To emphasize the lower fibers (from the center to the bottom of your bra line) of your chest, lie with your head at the lower end.

For Good Form and Safety:
• Make sure your wrists stay in line with your forearms.

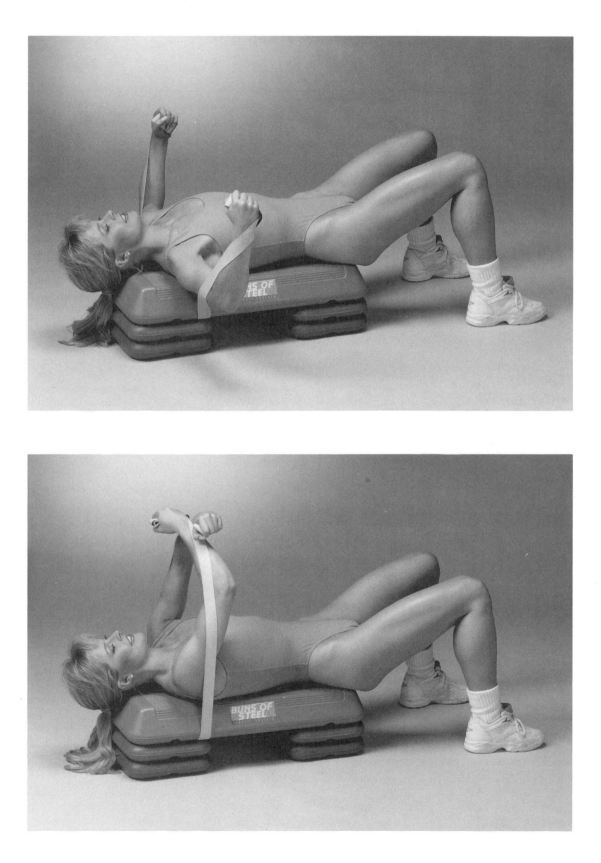

SHOULDERS

Exercise 7: SHOULDER PRESS

TARGET AREAS
Isolates your shoulder muscles.

The Setup: Sit on a chair with a dumbbell in each hand. Hold the dumbbells up at shoulder height slightly in front of your body with palms facing forward and your elbows pointing straight down toward the floor. Pull your abdominals inward and press firmly into the back of the chair while maintaining a natural arch in your lower back.

The Move:
• Exhale. Straighten your arms up over your head, gently squeezing your shoulder blades together as you go.
• Lightly touch the ends of the dumbbells together at the top of the movement.
• Inhale and return to the start.

Mind/Body Focus: As you're doing this exercise, imagine you're running your hands up and down an invisible wall. You're doing this right if you feel tension in the tops of your shoulders on the upward press.

Variations:
• If you find that one arm is noticeably weaker than the other, alternate one arm at a time. This allows you to give full attention to the form you're using with the weaker arm.
• To make this move more challenging and to focus on the form of one arm at a time, do all reps on one arm and then the other.
• Another way to increase the challenge of this exercise—as you lift the weights upward, rotate your palms so that they are facing behind you in the uppermost position. This will bring the back and sides of your shoulder muscles more into play.

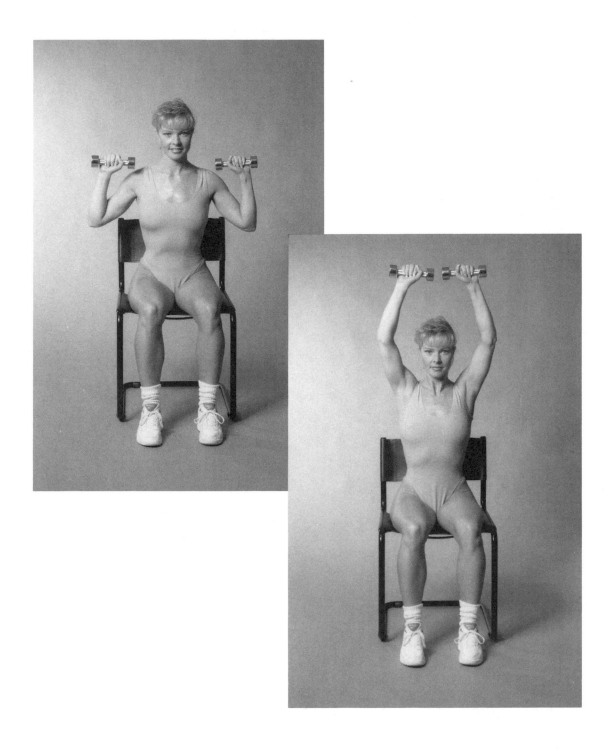

For Good Form and Safety:
• Don't drop your head forward or arch your back off the support. Concentrate on this especially as you lift the weights.

Exercise 8: LATERAL RAISE

TARGET AREAS
Target tones the shoulders.

The Setup: Stand with your knees slightly bent and your feet hip width apart. Grasp a dumbbell in each hand and hold them directly in front of the top of your thighs with your palms facing toward each other and your elbows slightly bent. Stand tall by pulling your abdominals inward and maintaining a natural curve in your spine.

The Move:
- Exhale. Keeping the slight bend in your elbows, raise the dumbbells up and out to the side until they reach shoulder height.
- Inhale. Slowly lower to the starting position.

Mind/Body Focus: Pretend you are pouring water from two large pitchers as your hands reach the top of the movement. The key to understanding this move is that your arms stay in one position and only your shoulders move. You'll feel tension in the sides of your shoulders as you lift the weight upward.

Variations:
- To increase the intensity of this move, sit on a chair or on a weight bench with back support. Start with your arms down at your sides.
- To bring the back of the shoulders into play, start and finish with your hands behind your lower back. You'll have to lean back from the waist and bend your knees for this version, but don't arch your lower back.

For Good Form and Safety:
- Be careful not to "rock" back and forth or arch your lower back. Keeping your knees slightly bent and your abdominals tight throughout will help.

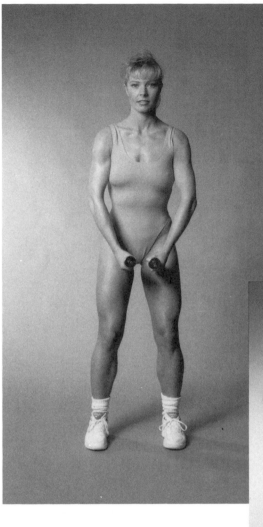

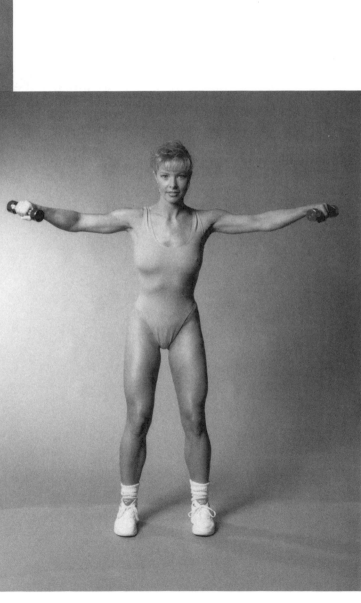

Exercise 9: UPRIGHT ROW WITH BAND

TARGET AREAS
Your shoulders, arms, and upper back.

The Setup: Stand with your feet hip width apart on the center of an exercise tube or band. Cross one end or handle of the band over the other. With your hands about an inch apart in front of your thighs and palms facing inward, hold one end or handle in each hand. Keep your elbows and knees slightly bent.

The Move:
• Exhale. Pull the handles up toward your chin by bending your elbows. The band will get tighter as you go. In the finished position your hands will be between your chest and your chin and your elbows will point out to the sides and slightly upward.
• Inhale and lower to the start.

Mind/Body Focus: Have you ever seen old movies of two men pumping the handles of a railroad car? That's exactly what this move should look like. If you do it correctly, you'll feel tension in the middle of your upper back and sides and backs of your shoulders as you pull upward.

Variations:
• Pull one arm upward at a time, then switch and perform an equal number of repetitions with the other arm.
• Alternate one arm at a time until you complete all reps with both arms.

For Good Form and Safety:
• Move your feet out to hip width position by first standing on the center of the band and then stepping one foot out to the side so that there is about six inches of band between your feet. This prevents the band from sliding out from under your feet.
• Standing tall with good posture will increase the effectiveness of this exercise.
• Pull the band up toward your chin rather than tilting your chin down to meet the band.

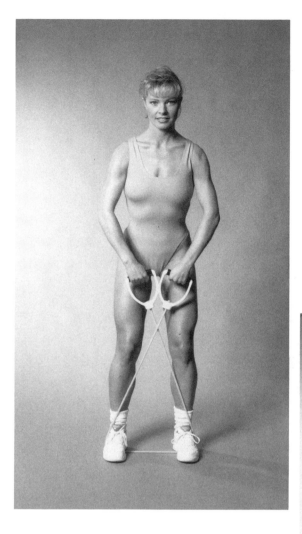

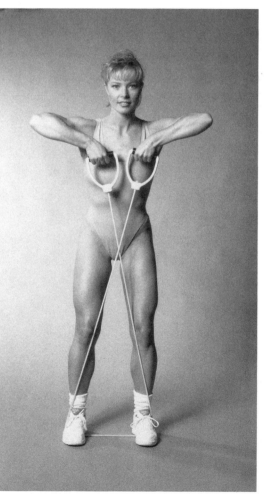

TRICEPS

Exercise 10: KICKBACK

TARGET AREAS
Isolates the backs of the upper arms, or triceps.

The Setup: Stand tall and bend your knees a few inches. Bend forward, *not by rounding your back*, but by bending at the hips. Hold a dumbbell in your left hand with your palm facing toward your body and place your right hand on top of your right thigh for support. With your elbow bent, bring your arm up so your elbow rests lightly against the side of your waist.

The Move:
• Straighten your forearm out behind you.
• Inhale and return to the starting position.
• Do the same number of repetitions with the other arm.

Mind/Body Focus: Think of your elbow joint as the hinge of a door, opening and closing. Keep your shoulder, upper arm, and elbow in place so that only your forearm moves. You'll feel the muscles in the back of your arm contracting as you extend your arm.

Variations:
• To involve even more of your triceps muscle in this move, twist as you extend your arm so that your palm is facing upward at the top of the movement.

For Good Form and Safety:
• Don't fully "lock out" your elbow at the top of the movement.
• To prevent your lower back from sagging, pull your abdominals inward and maintain a natural arch in your spine. By the same token, don't round your lower back upward, either.
• Keep your wrist in line with your forearm.

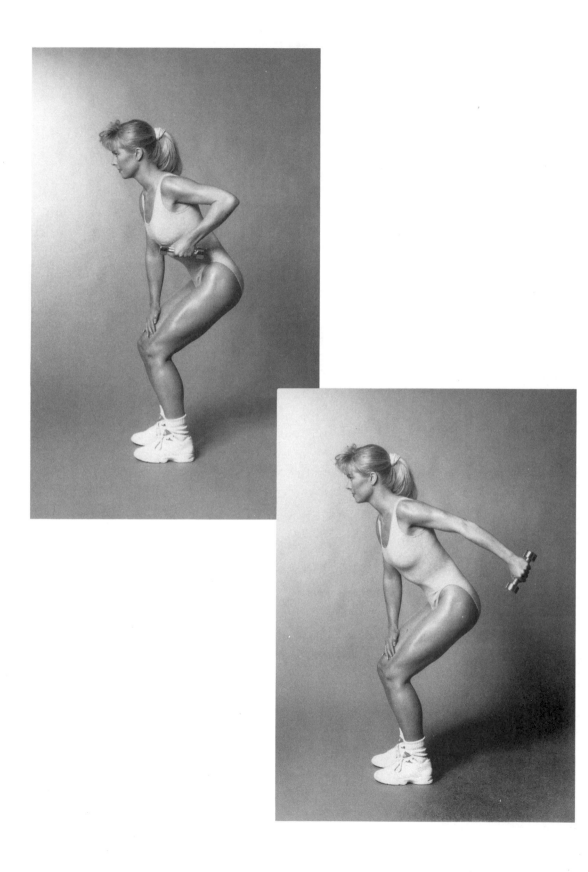

Exercise 11: TRICEPS EXTENSION WITH BAND

TARGET AREAS
Works the backs of the upper arms (triceps).

The Setup: Tie together the two ends of a small section of an exercise band or tube. Stand up tall with your feet hip width apart. While holding on to one end of the band with your right hand, place your right palm over the front of your left shoulder. Hold the other end of the band in your left hand with your palm facing inward. Bend your left elbow and hold it lightly against your side so that your hand is just in front of your waist.

The Move:
• Exhale. By passing your side, straighten your left arm out behind you so that the band gets tighter as you go.
• Inhale. Return to the start.
• Do an equal number of repetitions with the other arm.

Mind/Body Focus: The secret to this move is keeping your elbow still so that only your forearm moves. You're doing it right if you feel the muscles in the back of your upper arm working as you straighten out your arm.

Variations:
• To make this move more challenging, pulse one to two inches, eight to twelve times when your arm is in the straightened position.
• You can also add challenge to this move by increasing the range of motion. Rather than holding your working arm at your side, straighten it up directly over your shoulder. Then, bend your elbow and lower your forearm so that your hand touches the back of your shoulder and your elbow is pointing upward.

For Good Form and Safety:
• Make sure your wrist stays in line with the rest of your arm.
• Don't allow your elbow to fully lock in the finished position.

194

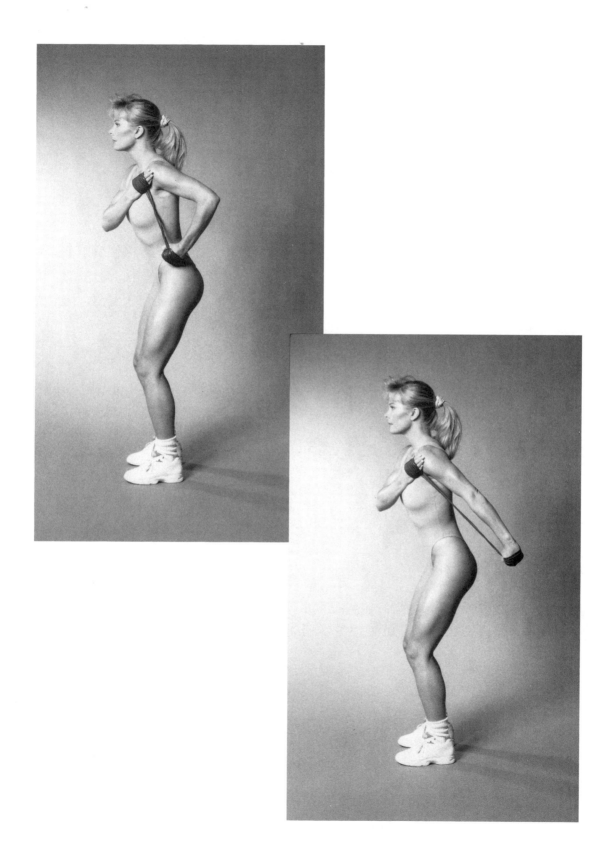

Biceps

Exercise 12: SEATED BICEPS CURL

TARGET AREAS
Target tones the fronts of your upper arms, or biceps.

The Setup: Sit on a chair with your feet hip width apart and flat on the floor. With your palms facing each other, hold a dumbbell in each hand. Let your arms hang down naturally at your sides.

The Move:
- Exhale. Bend both arms at the elbows and lift the weights up to shoulder level.
- As you bend your elbows, rotate your hands so that at the highest point your palms are facing your body.
- Inhale. Lower slowly to the start, rotating your hands back to the original position as you do so.

Mind/Body Focus: Picture each of your arms as a nutcracker. There's a nut placed in the well of your arm in front of your elbow joint, and you are trying to crack it open. You'll feel tension in the fronts of your upper arms as you lift the weights upward.

Variations:
- Do all repetitions with one arm and then the other.
- Eliminate the twist of your arm to place more emphasis on the outside of the upper arm and your wrist. In other words, in the topmost position, your thumb will be pointing back behind you.

For Good Form and Safety:
- Although you want to maintain a natural arch in your spine, avoid over-arching your lower back off the support. If this happens, there's a good chance you're using a weight that's too heavy or you're moving too quickly through the exercise.
- Once again, keep your wrist in line with the rest of your forearm.

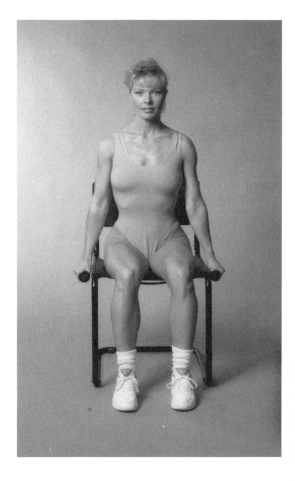

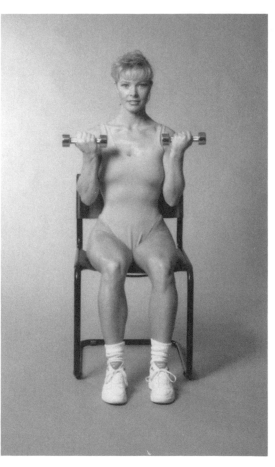

Exercise 13: STANDING BICEPS CURL WITH BAND

TARGET AREAS
Target tones the fronts of your upper arms (biceps).

The Setup: Stand on the center of an exercise tube or band with your feet hip width apart. With your arms down at your sides and your palms facing forward, hold a handle or end in each hand. Stand tall with your knees and elbows slightly bent and your abs tight.

The Move:
- Exhale. Bend your elbows, and curl both arms upward till your hands are in front of your shoulders. The band will be taut at the top of the movement.
- Inhale and lower slowly to the start.

Mind/Body Focus: Don't stop short of the top or bottom of this movement. A complete range of motion means raising your hands to shoulder height and then lowering slowly to the start so there is only a very slight bend in your elbows at the end of the movement. You're doing this right if you feel the muscles in the fronts of your upper arms contracting on the upward pull.

Variations:
- To make this exercise more challenging and focus on one arm at a time, alternate arms until you have completed all reps with both.
- To add even more challenge to this exercise and concentrate your efforts on one arm at a time, do all reps to one side and then the other.
- If you need more resistance, you can increase the tension of the band by stepping on it with one foot and holding both handles or ends in one hand.

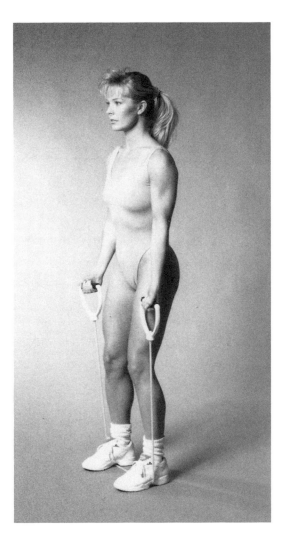

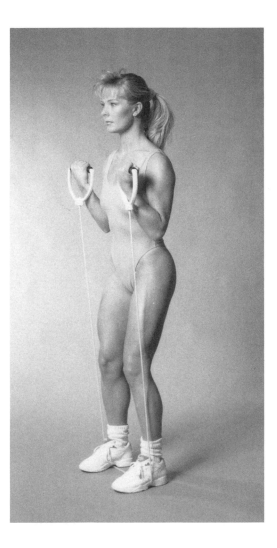

For Good Form and Safety:

- Keep your wrists aligned with your forearms and elbows close to—but not squeezing tightly into—your sides.
- To prevent the band from sliding out from underneath your feet when you first step on it, stand with both feet on the center of the band and then step one foot to the side so your feet are shoulder width apart and there is about six inches of band between your feet.

Upper Body Routines

Here are three upper body routines you can try. Choose the amount of time you want to spend target toning your upper body (ten, fifteen, or twenty minutes), then adapt that routine to your level. Once you've tried our routines for a while, you'll get a feel for which exercises you like best. When you feel comfortable, you can mix and match exercises to make up routines of your own as long as you remember to work from the largest to the smallest muscle groups. (First the upper back, then chest, shoulders, triceps, biceps—follow the order they're listed in the chapter.)

Equipment you'll need: A step with three to four sets of risers, one or more sets of dumbbells, exercise band or tube, a chair.

How Many Reps Should I Do?

Do eight to fifteen repetitions each set. When you can do fifteen repetitions easily and with good form, move on to a more difficult variation of that exercise the next time you work out. If you find it difficult to do at least eight repetitions while maintaining good form, try an easier version of the exercise.

How Much Weight Should I Use?

Don't be afraid of using weights that feel heavy when you do these upper body exercises. Using resistance (dumbbells or an exercise band) that allows you to complete eight to fifteen repetitions with proper form will give you upper body tone and definition, *not bulk.* If you don't feel it when you work it, you won't see the results in the mirror. Increase the weight when you can do fifteen reps easily and with good form; if you can't get through at least eight reps, decrease the weight or try an easier variation.

For beginners, three- to eight-pound dumbbells should be enough resistance to start with in these exercises. Intermediates, you'll probably need five- to twelve-pound dumbbells. For advanced target toners, eight- to twenty-pound dumbbells should be sufficient resistance.

More than likely you'll find that you can handle a lot more weight in some exercises than in others. In general you'll use heavier weights when you perform exercises with the larger muscle groups such as your back, chest, and shoulders and lighter weights when you do exercises for the smaller muscle groups of your arms. You may have to do a bit of experimentation to determine the amount of resistance you need for each particular exercise.

How Much Should I Rest Between Sets?

Rest from thirty to ninety seconds between each exercise set. This will allow your muscles enough time to recover so they are strong enough to work their hardest when you do the next set but will not be so long that you lose the intensity and focus of your workout. You'll find that as you become stronger, you won't need as much rest between sets.

How Often Should I Target Tone My Upper Body?

For best results, target tone your upper body two to three times a week with at least one day of rest in between each workout session.

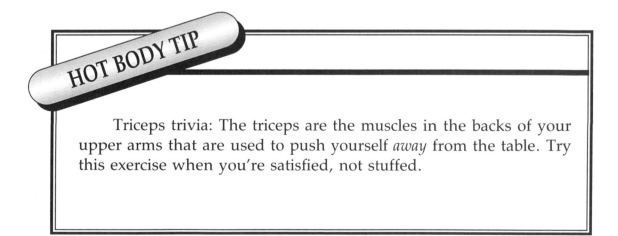

HOT BODY TIP

Triceps trivia: The triceps are the muscles in the backs of your upper arms that are used to push yourself *away* from the table. Try this exercise when you're satisfied, not stuffed.

Upper Body Isolation Routines

10-Minute Routine

(Beginner)

ORDER	EXERCISE	RESISTANCE/VARIATION	SETS
1	Pullover	Dumbbell	1
2	Lat Pulldown with Band	Exercise band	1
3	Push-up	None	1
4	Chest fly	Dumbbells	1
5	Shoulder Press	Dumbbells	1
6	Kickback	Dumbbell	1
7	Seated Biceps Curl	Dumbbells	1

(Intermediate)

ORDER	EXERCISE	RESISTANCE/VARIATION	SETS
1	Pullover	Dumbbell	1
2	Lat Pulldown with Band	Exercise band	1
3	Push-up	None	1
4	Chest Fly	Dumbbells	1
5	Shoulder Press	Dumbbells; alternate arms	1
6	Kickback	Dumbbell	1
7	Seated Biceps Curl	Dumbbells; alternate arms	1

(ADVANCED)

ORDER	EXERCISE	RESISTANCE/VARIATION	SETS
1	Pullover	Dumbbell	1
2	Lat Pulldown with Band	Exercise band	1
3	Push-up	None	1
4	Chest Fly	Dumbbells; incline	1
5	Shoulder Press	Dumbbells; alternate arms	1
6	Kickback	Dumbbell; with twist	1
7	Seated Biceps Curl	Dumbbells; alternate arms	1

HOT BODY TIP

Cellulite is no different from any other type of body fat except that it seems harder to lose. Target toning, aerobic exercise, and a sensible, low-fat diet will make a difference. Eat plenty of fiber and limit consumption of alcohol, caffeine, and processed foods.

HOT BODY TIP

Do something for the environment as well as your waistline. Walk, jog, or skate to the corner store instead of taking the car. That ten-minute trip to pick up a carton of milk can burn nearly one hundred calories.

15-Minute Routine

(Beginner)

ORDER	EXERCISE	RESISTANCE/VARIATION	SETS
1	Seated Row	Exercise band	1
2	Lat Pulldown with Band	Exercise band	1
3	Push-up	None	1
4	Chest Fly	Dumbbells	2
5	Shoulder Press	Dumbbells	1
6	Lateral Raise	Dumbbells	1
7	Triceps Extension with Band	Exercise band	1
8	Seated Biceps Curl	Dumbbells	1

(Intermediate)

ORDER	EXERCISE	RESISTANCE/VARIATION	SETS
1	Seated Row	Exercise band	1
2	Lat Pulldown with Band	Exercise band; all reps to one side	1
3	Push-up	None	1
4	Chest Fly	Dumbbells; one set on incline	2
5	Shoulder Press	Dumbbells; alternate arms	1
6	Lateral Raise	Dumbbells	1
7	Triceps Extension with Band	Exercise band	1
8	Seated Biceps Curl	Dumbbells; alternate arms	1

(ADVANCED)

ORDER	EXERCISE	RESISTANCE/VARIATION	SETS
1	Seated Row	Exercise band; single arm	1
2	Lat Pulldown with Band	Exercise band; all reps to one side	1
3	Push-up	Add band	1
4	Chest Fly	Dumbbells; one set on incline	2
5	Shoulder Press	Dumbbells; add rotation	1
6	Lateral Raise	Dumbbells; seated	1
7	Triceps Extension with Band	Exercise band; overhead	1
8	Seated Biceps Curl	Dumbbells; alternate arms	1

HOT BODY TIP

If you eat one hundred fewer calories per day and burn off an extra one hundred calories per day, you can shed up to twenty pounds a year. (That's the equivalent of one less pat of butter and a daily ten-minute target toning session.)

HOT BODY TIP

Another nutrition myth: You'll gain more weight if you eat right before bedtime. Recent studies have shown that if your calorie intake and activity level remain the same, you won't store a significantly higher number of food calories as fat as you slumber even if you eat a full meal before you hit the hay. The calories you consume will simply be burned when needed.

20-Minute Routine

(Beginner)

ORDER	EXERCISE	RESISTANCE/VARIATION	SETS
1	Pullover	Dumbbell	1
2	Lat Pulldown	Exercise band	1
3	Seated Row with Band	Exercise band	1
4	Push-up	None	1
5	Chest Fly	Dumbbells	1
6	Crossover with Band	Exercise band; bench press only	1
7	Shoulder Press	Dumbbells	1
8	Upright Row with Band	Exercise band	1
9	Kickback	Dumbbell	2
10	Standing Biceps Curl with Band	Exercise band	1

(Intermediate)

ORDER	EXERCISE	RESISTANCE/VARIATION	SETS
1	Pullover	Dumbbell	1
2	Seated Row with Band	Exercise band; one set with single arm	2
3	Push-up	None	1
4	Chest Fly	Dumbbells; one incline, one decline	1
5	Crossover with Band	Exercise band	1
6	Shoulder Press	Dumbbells	1
7	Upright Row with Band	Exercise band	1
8	Kickback	Dumbbell; add twist	2
9	Standing Biceps Curl with Band	Exercise band	1

(ADVANCED)

ORDER	EXERCISE	RESISTANCE/VARIATION	SETS
1	Pullover	Dumbbell	1
2	Seated Row with Band	Exercise band; one set with single arm	2
3	Push-up	Exercise band	1
4	Chest Fly	Dumbbells; one incline, one decline	1
5	Crossover with Band	Exercise band	1
6	Shoulder Press	Dumbbells; add rotation	1
7	Upright Row with Band	Exercise band	1
8	Kickback	Dumbbell; add twist	2
9	Standing Biceps Curl with Band	Exercise band; both handles in one hand	1

HOT BODY TIP

Treat injuries and muscle soreness with R.I.C.E.: rest, ice, compression, and elevation.

HOT BODY TIP

Wearing three-inch heels puts 76 percent more pressure on the ball of the foot than going barefoot; a two-inch heel, 57 percent more pressure. This extra stress on the foot and your entire body alignment may lead to foot abnormalities, calf strains, and lower back pain. Wear flats when you can, and if you must wear heels, stretch out your feet and calves frequently.

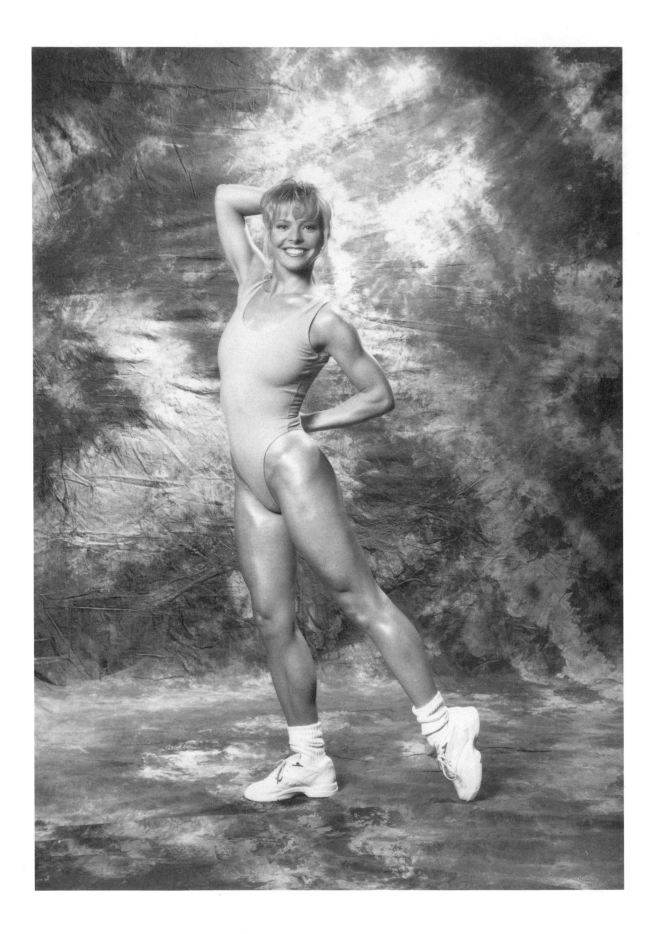

CHAPTER 10

Putting It All Together: Total-Body Routines

Now that you've got a taste of what target toning can do for you, it's time to put it all together. This chapter will show you how to spice up your training by adding some variety to the mix. Using these specialized Buns of Steel techniques will allow you to adapt your workouts for any situation, mood, or preference.

The process of reshaping your body takes time, and maintaining your ideal body is an ongoing process. By keeping your workouts fresh and exciting, you'll always look forward to doing them. And your body can always use a change. Sometimes doing something a little differently will be just the thing to take you to the next level.

Luckily you've got plenty of options with the Buns of Steel Total-Body Workout. In this chapter you'll learn some of the different techniques and styles you can use to put the spark back into your workouts. Even if you're not interested in changing things around just yet, read on. You'll also learn about adapting your Buns of Steel program for travel, the gym, and when you're tight on time.

Actually, the routines that follow are optional. You may be perfectly happy to firm up your buns, chisel definition into your thighs, or work toward any other target toning goal by sticking with the routines in the back of each target toning chapter. If that's the case, go for it! But if you get the urge to try something new, these workouts are perfect for putting a little different spin on the concept of target toning.

Whole-Body Training

Your natural impulse will be to give more of your attention to the areas of your body you feel need the most work. By all means, use the target toning routines outlined in the back of each chapter to take aim at your trouble zones, but remember—for the total picture, you're going to need to give at least some attention to all the muscles in your body if your goal is to sculpt a well-balanced, proportioned physique. (And we know it is!)

If you have time, you can do one routine from the back of each chapter for a complete total-body workout. But you may not always have an hour or more to catch a workout. That's where whole-body target toning comes in. Decide how much total time you want to spend target toning your entire body (fifteen, twenty, or twenty-five minutes), then adapt the routines that follow to your level.

What if you travel a lot or you're planning a vacation? Then take special note of the twenty-minute routine that follows. We designed this routine especially to be taken on the road. You can do it anywhere. The only equipment needed is an exercise band or tube, a particularly versatile form of resistance that's light and fits easily into any purse or suitcase. As for the exercises in this routine that call for a step, it usually isn't too hard to find a suitable substitute. Use your imagination. You can do calf raises off the edge of a staircase, for instance, or standing on top of a thick telephone book propped against the wall so it doesn't slide around. Crossovers can be done lying on the floor with your head, neck, and shoulders propped up on a couple of pillows.

The Method:
• These exercises work your muscles from the largest to the smallest. Do them in the order listed.

210

• Do eight to fifteen repetitions each set. If you can't do eight with good form, decrease the weight. If you can do fifteen reps easily and with good form, up the weight the next workout.

• Rest thirty to ninety seconds between sets. As you get stronger, you won't need to rest as much.

• Be sure to include the complete warm-up and cooldown described on pages 26 and 33 before and after doing one of these whole-body routines.

Whole-Body Routines

15-Minute Routine (Beginner)

ORDER	EXERCISE	RESISTANCE/VARIATION	SETS	PAGE NUMBER
1	Squat	None	1	60
2	Hip Press	None	1	96
3	Tilt and Squeeze	None	1	102
4	One Leg Quad Pulse	None	1	120
5	Step and Curl	None	1	126
6	Standing Calf Raise off Step	None	1	132
7	Pullover	Dumbbell	1	174
8	Push-up	None	1	180
9	Shoulder Press	Dumbbells	1	186
10	Kickback	Dumbbell	1	192
11	Seated Biceps Curl	Dumbbells	1	196
12	Basic Crunch	None	1	148

15-Minute Routine (Intermediate)

ORDER	EXERCISE	RESISTANCE/VARIATION	SETS	PAGE NUMBER
1	Squat	Dumbbells	1	60
2	Hip Press	Exercise band	1	96
3	Tilt and Squeeze	None	1	102
4	One Leg Quad Pulse	None	1	120
5	Step and Curl	Dumbbells	1	126
6	Standing Calf Raise off Step	Dumbbell	1	132
7	Pullover	Dumbbell	1	174
8	Push-up	None	1	180
9	Shoulder Press	Dumbbells	1	186
10	Kickback	Dumbbell	1	192
11	Seated Biceps Curl	Dumbbells	1	196
12	Basic Crunch	None	1	148

HOT BODY TIP

Don't skip a meal to "save up calories" for tonight's big feast or you may wind up so hungry that you can't resist pigging out. Always eat a healthy breakfast and lunch, and if you're attending a late evening function, avoid a binge by having a low-fat snack beforehand. Some good choices are air-popped popcorn, fruit, or low-fat yogurt.

15-MINUTE ROUTINE (ADVANCED)

ORDER	EXERCISE	RESISTANCE/VARIATION	SETS	PAGE NUMBER
1	Squat	Dumbbells	1	60
2	Hip Press	Exercise band	1	96
3	Tilt and Squeeze	Ball	1	102
4	One Leg Quad Pulse	None	1	120
5	Step and Curl	Dumbbells	1	126
6	Standing Calf Raise off Step	Dumbbell	1	132
7	Pullover	Dumbbell	1	174
8	Push-up	None	1	180
9	Shoulder Press	Dumbbell—add rotation	1	186
10	Kickback	Dumbbell—add twist	1	192
11	Seated Biceps Curl	Dumbbell	1	196
12	Total Crunch	None	1	152

HOT BODY TIP

You're never too old to target tone! Recent studies have shown that people in their eighties gain the same percentage of strength from regular workouts as people in their twenties.

HOT BODY TIP

Exercising with a partner may help keep you on track. You can encourage and push each other. Besides, it may be one of the most inexpensive forms of therapy going! Share your ideas and worries during a workout with a person you trust.

20-MINUTE ROUTINE (BEGINNER)

ORDER	EXERCISE	RESISTANCE/ VARIATION	SETS	PAGE NUMBER
1	Squat Pulse	None	2	64
2	Plié	None	1	62
3	Hip Press	Exercise band	1	96
4	Supported Inner Thigh Lift	None	1	100
5	Standing Leg Extension with Band	Exercise band	1	122
6	Standing Leg Curl with Band	Exercise band	1	128
7	Standing Calf Raise off Step	None	1	132
8	Lat Pulldown with Band	Exercise band	1	178
9	Crossover with Band	Exercise band—Chest Press version	1	184
10	Upright Row with Band	Exercise band	1	190
11	Triceps Extension with Band	Exercise band	1	194
12	Standing Biceps Curl with Band	Exercise band	1	198
13	Abdominal Grounding	None	1	146
14	Basic Crunch	None	1	148
15	Crossover Crunch	None	1	150

HOT BODY TIP

Moisturizer is a must to keep skin from drying out, but don't put it on right before a workout. Even light moisturizers will mix with sweat to clog pores, leading to rashes, acne, and other skin conditions. And since moisture is the key to silky-smooth skin, drink at least eight glasses of water a day.

20-MINUTE ROUTINE (INTERMEDIATE)

ORDER	EXERCISE	RESISTANCE/VARIATION	SETS	PAGE NUMBER
1	Squat Pulse	None	2	64
2	Plié	None	1	62
3	Penguins	Exercise band	1	94
4	Glute Raise with Crossover	None	1	104
5	Standing Leg Extension with Band	Exercise band	1	122
6	Standing Leg Curl with Band	Exercise band	1	128
7	Standing Calf Raise off Step	None	1	132
8	Seated Row with Band	Exercise band	1	176
9	Crossover with Band	Exercise band	1	184
10	Upright Row with Band	Exercise band	1	190
11	Triceps Extension with Band	Exercise band	1	194
12	Standing Biceps Curl with Band	Exercise band	1	198
13	Abdominal Grounding	None	1	146
14	Basic Crunch	None	1	148
15	Crossover Crunch	None	1	150

HOT BODY TIP

Chose an exercise intensity to fit your mood. For example, if you're frustrated, try a fast-paced workout to help calm yourself down. If you've got things on your mind, a moderate-paced workout will help you relax and think better.

20-Minute Routine (Advanced)

ORDER	EXERCISE	RESISTANCE/VARIATION	SETS	PAGE NUMBER
1	Squat Pulse	None	2	64
2	Plié	None	1	62
3	Penguins	Exercise band—hold for a count of five at the top	1	94
4	Glute Raise with Crossover	None	1	104
5	Standing Leg Extension with Band	Exercise band	1	122
6	Standing Leg Curl with Band	Exercise band—pulse eight times at the top	1	128
7	Standing Calf Raise off Step	None—work one leg at a time	1	132
8	Seated Row with Band	Exercise band—work one arm at a time	1	176
9	Crossover with Band	Exercise band—incline bench	1	184
10	Lateral Raise	Dumbbells	1	188
11	Triceps Extension with Band	Exercise band	1	194
12	Standing Biceps Curl with Band	Exercise band	1	198
13	Abdominal Grounding	None	1	146
14	Crunch and Pulse	None	1	154
15	Crossover Crunch	None	1	150

25-MINUTE ROUTINE (BEGINNER)

ORDER	EXERCISE	RESISTANCE/VARIATION	SETS	PAGE NUMBER
1	Squat	None	1	60
2	3-D Lunge	None	1	70
3	Kneeling Glute Raise with Band	Exercise band	1	80
4	Hip Press	None	1	96
5	Side Lying Outward Rotation	None	1	98
6	Supported Inner Thigh Lift	None	1	100
7	Kneeling Glute Raise with Band	None	1	80
8	Bump Squat	None	1	124
9	Step and Curl	None	1	126
10	Standing Calf Raise off Step	None	1	132
11	Abdominal Grounding	None	1	146
12	Total Crunch	None	1	152
13	Crossover Crunch	None	1	150
14	Incline Reverse Curl	Decline version	1	160
15	Pullover	Dumbbell	1	174
16	Crossover with Band	Exercise band	1	184
17	Shoulder Press	Dumbbells	1	186
18	Triceps Extension with Band	Exercise band	1	194
19	Standing Biceps Curl with Band	Exercise band		198

25-Minute Routine (Intermediate)

ORDER	EXERCISE	RESISTANCE/VARIATION	SETS	PAGE NUMBER
1	Squat	Dumbbells	1	60
2	3-D Lunge	None	1	70
3	Kneeling Glute Raise with Band	Pulse at top	1	80
4	Hip Press	Exercise band	1	96
5	Side Lying Outward Rotation	None	1	98
6	Supported Inner Thigh Lift	None	1	100
7	Kneeling Glute Raise with Band	Alternate with upward press	1	80
8	Bump Squat	None	1	124
9	Step and Curl	Dumbbells	1	126
10	Standing Calf Raise off Step	Dumbbells	1	132
11	Abdominal Grounding	None	1	146
12	Total Crunch	None	1	152
13	Circular Crunch	None	1	156
14	Reverse Curl	None	1	158
15	Pullover	Dumbbell	1	174
16	Crossover with Band	Exercise band	1	184
17	Shoulder Press	Dumbbells—alternate	1	187
18	Triceps Extension with Band	Exercise band	1	194
19	Standing Biceps Curl with Band	Exercise band		198

25-MINUTE ROUTINE (ADVANCED)

ORDER	EXERCISE	RESISTANCE/VARIATION	SETS	PAGE NUMBER
1	Squat	Dumbbells	1	60
2	3-D Lunge	None	1	70
3	Kneeling Glute Raise with Band	Pulse at top	1	80
4	Hip Press	Exercise band	1	96
5	Side Lying Outward Rotation	Ankle weight	1	98
6	Supported Inner Thigh Lift	Ankle weight	1	100
7	Kneeling Glute Raise with Band	Alternate with upward press	1	80
8	Bump Squat	On toes	1	124
9	Step and Curl	Dumbbells	1	126
10	Standing Calf Raise off Step	Dumbbell—single leg	1	132
11	Abdominal Grounding	None	1	146
12	Total Crunch	None	1	152
13	Circular Crunch	None	1	156
14	Incline Reverse Curl	None	1	160
15	Pullover	Dumbbells	1	174
16	Crossover with Band	Exercise band	1	184
17	Shoulder Press	Dumbbells—alternate	1	187
18	Triceps Extension with Band	Exercise band—press upward	1	194
19	Standing Biceps Curl with Band	Exercise band—both handles in one hand	1	198

Split Routines

Some days you just don't have an hour or more to spend on a workout. Does that mean you should give up the idea of training altogether? Of course not! That's not a Buns of Steel attitude! You can still get in a full-body workout by working different muscles on alternate days. This is a Buns of Steel technique we refer to as a **split routine.** Splitting up your routine so that you do half your training on one day and half the next is ideal if you have only a little time here or there but you're still determined to do a complete workout. It's just as effective as doing all your exercises on the same day, so don't worry about compromising your results.

We've developed some quick split routines for you to try when you're really pressed for time. You can get by with as little as five minutes of target toning a day. *Any amount of time* you spend target toning is time well spent.

The Method:
• Alternate day 1 and day 2 of each split routine. Do each workout two to three times a week for a total of four to six workouts.

• As always, do eight to fifteen repetitions each set. If you can't do eight with good form, decrease the weight. If you can do fifteen reps easily and with good form, up the weight the next workout.

• Take as little rest as you need—at least thirty seconds between sets, but no more than ninety seconds.

• If you find that the idea of splitting up your routines works well for you, then try making up some of your own. For best results, make sure each muscle group gets exercised at least twice a week. Most people will see noticeable results after six to eight weeks of this type of training.

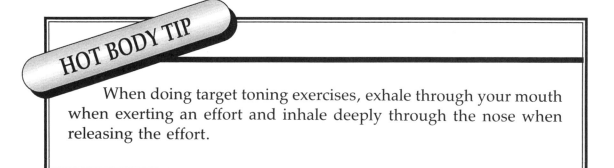

HOT BODY TIP

When doing target toning exercises, exhale through your mouth when exerting an effort and inhale deeply through the nose when releasing the effort.

5-Minute-a-Day Split Routine (Beginner)

DAY 1 (BUNS, INNER/OUTER THIGHS, LEGS)

ORDER	EXERCISE	RESISTANCE/VARIATION	SETS	PAGE NUMBER
1	Squat	None	1	60
2	Outward Step and Squat	None	1	92
3	Supported Inner Thigh Lift	None	1	100
4	One Leg Quad Pulse	None	1	120
5	Step and Curl	None	1	126

Advanced and Intermediate: Add dumbbells to Squat, Outward Step and Squat, and Step and Curl. *Advanced:* Add ankle weight to Supported Inner Thigh Lift; lower into Squat for One Leg Quad Pulse.

DAY 2 (UPPER BODY, ABDOMINALS)

ORDER	EXERCISE	RESISTANCE/VARIATION	SETS	PAGE NUMBER
1	Pullover	Dumbbell	1	174
2	Push-up	None	1	180
3	Shoulder Press	Dumbbell	1	186
4	Basic Crunch	None	1	148
5	Reverse Curl	None	1	158

Advanced and Intermediate: Hold five counts at top of Basic Crunch. *Advanced:* Add exercise band to Reverse Curl.

HOT BODY TIP

Time-saver: There's a common notion that you should work your abdominal muscles every day, but most experts agree they should be worked three times a week just like any other muscle group. Not only will you find it's more effective to work your abs less, you'll also have more time to spend target toning other muscles!

10-Minute-a-Day Split Routine (Intermediate and Advanced)

Day 1 (Buns, Inner/Outer Thighs, Legs)

ORDER	EXERCISE	RESISTANCE/VARIATION	SETS	PAGE NUMBER
1	Squat	Dumbbells	1	60
2	Basic Lunge	Dumbbells	1	68
3	Penguins	Exercise band; hold at top 5 counts	1	94
4	Side Lying Outward Rotation	Ankle weight	1	98
5	Glute Raise with Crossover	None	1	104
6	Inner Thigh Press-Out	Exercise band above knees	1	106
7	Standing Leg Extension with Band	Exercise band	1	122
8	Step and Curl	Dumbbells	1	126
9	Standing Calf Raise off Step	Dumbbell	1	132

Beginner: Omit dumbbells where listed. Omit five-count hold on Penguins and band on Inner Thigh Press-Out.

HOT BODY TIP

Too little is not enough. Eating fewer than 1,200 calories per day puts your body into starvation mode. Your metabolism will slow down, which means you'll burn fewer calories and have a harder time losing weight and keeping it off. On the other hand, regular exercise is the best way to rev up your metabolism and keep your internal furnace stoked.

DAY 2 (UPPER BODY, ABDOMINALS)

ORDER	EXERCISE	RESISTANCE/VARIATION	SETS	PAGE NUMBER
1	Seated Row with Band	Exercise band	1	176
2	Lat Pulldown with Band	Exercise band	1	178
3	Chest Fly	Dumbbells; 2nd set on incline	2	182
4	Upright Row with Band	Exercise band	1	190
5	Kickback	Dumbbell; rotate hand	1	192
6	Standing Biceps Curl with Band	Exercise band; one hand version	1	198
7	Circular Crunch	None	1	156
8	Incline Reverse Curl	None	1	160

Beginner: Omit incline on second set of Chest Fly; omit hand rotation on Kickback; do standard version of Standing Biceps Curl with Band. Substitute Crossover Crunch for Circular Crunch and Reverse Curl for Incline Reverse Curl.

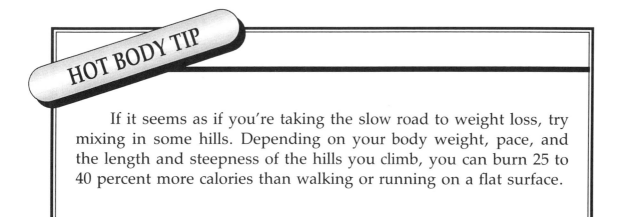

HOT BODY TIP

If it seems as if you're taking the slow road to weight loss, try mixing in some hills. Depending on your body weight, pace, and the length and steepness of the hills you climb, you can burn 25 to 40 percent more calories than walking or running on a flat surface.

Fat Burner Circuits

It's true that building muscle through target toning speeds up your metabolism and results in a higher calorie burn throughout the day. However, target toning sessions alone aren't usually enough to burn a lot of calories the way aerobic activities do. One way to turn a strength training session into a fat-burning workout is with **circuit training,** a method of target toning that involves doing all your exercises in quick succession with no rest in between.

Try a circuit training session if you're looking for something a little different or you really want to work up a good sweat.

The Setup: Before you start your circuit training workout, gather together everything you need. In the sample circuit we've designed for you below, you'll need one or more sets of dumbbells, an exercise band or tube, and a step.

The Method:
• Do a set of eight to fifteen repetitions of a target training move and then move immediately to the next set. Don't take any rest in between sets. Move quickly from one move to the next.

• Use slightly less resistance or an easier version of each target toning exercise than you usually do. (For instance, if you normally hold dumbbells while doing squats, try doing them with a lighter weight or no weight at all.)

• Move through the workout in the order of exercises given.

• Notice that the routine we've designed for you intersperses upper body and abdominal exercises between exercises for the buns, legs, and inner and outer thighs. That's so you don't tire one muscle group too quickly. When you've had more experience with circuit training, you can design one of your own to focus on a single body part or just a few areas.

SAMPLE CIRCUIT FOR TOTAL BODY

ORDER	EXERCISE	RESISTANCE/VARIATION	SETS	PAGE NUMBER
1	Squat	None	1	60
2	Jumpers	None	1	76
3	Basic Crunch	None	1	148
4	Penguins	Exercise band	1	94
5	Supported Inner Thigh Lift	None	1	100
6	Reverse Curl	None	1	158
7	Lat Pulldown with Band	Exercise band	1	178
8	Wall Sit	None; 15 seconds	1	118
9	Standing Leg Curl with Band	Exercise band	1	128
10	Chest Fly	Dumbbells	1	182
11	Standing Calf Raise off Step	None	1	132
12	Lateral Raise	Dumbbells	1	188
13	Crossover Crunch	None	1	150
14	Triceps Extension with Band	Exercise band	1	194
15	Standing Biceps Curl with Band	Exercise band	1	198
16	Squat and Lift	None	1	72

Beginner and Intermediate: Do it once all the way through (15 minutes). *Advanced:* Go for it! Do it twice all the way through (30 minutes).

Supercircuit

The idea behind **supercircuit** training is much the same as basic circuit training—to introduce an aerobic element into your target toning workouts. The supercircuit goes one step beyond by including an interval of aerobic exercise between each set of target toning exercises.

Adding one supercircuit a week into your exercise schedule is a good way to shake up your training regimen when you're bored, and it's a perfect alternative when you don't have time to squeeze in your normal aerobic workout and target toning routine.

The Setup: Before you start your supercircuit, gather together everything you need. In the sample supercircuit we've designed for you below, you'll need a stopwatch or clock with a second hand, one or more sets of dumbbells, a step, and a chair or weight bench.

The Method:
• Alternate sets of eight to fifteen repetitions of a target training move with a timed interval of an aerobic activity such as the stationary bike, jogging or marching in place, a stair climber, or jump rope. Start your supercircuit with a resistance training exercise interval.

• Don't take any rest in between your cardiovascular set and your target toning set. Move quickly from one thing to the next.

• Do your cardiovascular work with a slightly stronger intensity than usual, and use slightly less resistance or an easier version of each target toning exercise than usual. (For instance, if you normally add pulse to your bun sweeps, do the basic version instead.)

• Notice that in this routine you do a lower body target toning exercise, and then the next target toning exercise you do is for the upper or middle body. That's so you don't tire one set of muscles too quickly and to ensure that blood flows to every part of your body. When you've had more experience with supercircuit training, you can design one of your own to focus on a single body part or just a few areas.

SAMPLE SUPERCIRCUIT FOR TOTAL BODY

ORDER	EXERCISE	RESISTANCE/VARIATION	SETS	PAGE NUMBER
1	Total Crunch	None	1	152
2	Squat	None	1	60
3	Pullover	Dumbbell	1	174
4	Outward Step and Squat	None	1	92
5	Push-up	None	1	180
6	Inner Thigh Press-Out	None	1	106
7	Shoulder Press	Dumbbells	1	186
8	Bump Squat	None	1	124
9	Kickback	Dumbbell	1	192
10	Step and Curl	None	1	126
11	Standing Calf Raise off Step	None	1	132
12	Seated Biceps Curl	Dumbbells	1	196

Beginner: Do 30 seconds on stationary bike, stair climber, step, jump rope, jogging, or marching in place between target toning sets (18 minutes). *Intermediate:* Do 45 seconds of one of the aforementioned aerobic activities between target toning sets (21 minutes). *Advanced:* Do 60 seconds of one of the aforementioned cardiovascular activities between target sets (24 minutes).

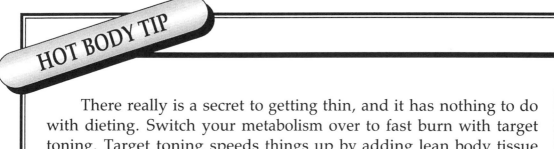

HOT BODY TIP

There really is a secret to getting thin, and it has nothing to do with dieting. Switch your metabolism over to fast burn with target toning. Target toning speeds things up by adding lean body tissue (muscle) to your body. This will help you burn extra fat and calories even when you're not exercising.

Superadvanced Body Blaster Techniques

Okay, you've been training for a while and you're all revved up. Sure, the routines at the end of each chapter have gotten you results, but you're feeling amazingly strong, ready for action. What you need is a longer, more intense target toning routine, or what we call a **body blaster.**

Body blaster routines are for intermediate and advanced exercisers. You should train consistently for a month or more before you try one. Body blasters use all the same exercises we've shown you in the chapters, but you'll do more of them and you'll combine them in ways that intensify each move.

If you decide to do a body blaster routine, allot yourself a little more time. The sample routine below takes about forty-five minutes to get through. Don't do more than one body blaster routine a week. They're meant to interject some very high intensity training into your normal routine, but overdoing them may lead to overtraining and a risk of injury—too much of a good thing!

Before you check out the sample body blaster routine, take some time to study these three advanced techniques you'll be using: supersets, pyramids, and negatives. We've developed these techniques to help you chisel and define your body into steely perfection. (You may want to incorporate one or more of them into your normal target training.)

Superset: A combination of two sets of two different exercises with no rest in between. The most intense form of supersetting involves pairing two exercises that work the same muscle, like the squat and squat pulse pairing in the sample routine below. This is a great way to stimulate any especially stubborn trouble zone. You can also superset two muscle groups that have opposing actions like the front of your thigh and the back of your thigh or the front of your arm and the back of your arm.

Even though you'll take little or no rest between the exercises in a superset, be sure to take your normal thirty- to ninety-second rest between a superset and the next set you do.

Pyramids: Involves making each set of an exercise progressively harder. One way to do this is to add more weight with each new set; in general you should use the next heaviest weight as you pyramid upward. When doing the three chest fly sets listed in the sample routine below, you might do the first one with five-pound dumbbells, the second set with eight, and the third set with ten.

Some people prefer doing descending pyramids by starting with a heavier weight and using a lighter weight each set. It's okay to pyramid this way if you feel more comfortable. You'll still get the same results.

Negatives: That's where you give equal time to both the up and the down phase of an exercise. Say you're doing the negative version of the basic crunch in the sample routine. Normally you would place emphasis on curling your head, neck, and shoulders off the floor and then relax as you return to your starting position. But when doing the negative basic crunch, you'll slow down the lowering phase of the exercise and concentrate on tightening your muscles on the way down. If you have a training partner, she can put gentle pressure on your shoulders for you to resist against.

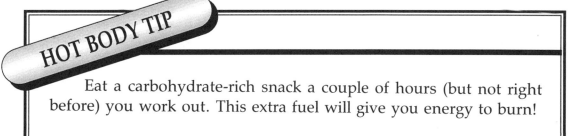

HOT BODY TIP

Eat a carbohydrate-rich snack a couple of hours (but not right before) you work out. This extra fuel will give you energy to burn!

HOT BODY TIP

Exercise in disguise: Take the stairs instead of the elevator, park your car at the far end of the parking lot, and stand when you're on a phone call. These small extra efforts can add up to increased muscle tone and more calories burned.

SAMPLE BODY BLASTER ROUTINE

ORDER	EXERCISE	RESISTANCE	TECHNIQUE	SETS	PAGE NUMBER
1	Squat plus Squat Pulse	None	Superset	2	60, 64
2	3-D Lunge	None	Basic Version	1	70
3	Side Lying Outward Rotation plus Supported Inner Thigh Lift (do both with right leg, then with left)	Ankle weight	Superset	1	98, 100
4	One Leg Quad Pulse	None	Negative	2	120
5	Step and Curl	Dumbbells	Basic Version	2	126
6	Standing Calf Raise off Step plus Seated Calf Raise	None	Superset	1	132, 134
7	Abdominal Grounding	None	Basic Version	1	146
8	Basic Crunch	None	Negative	1	148
9	Reverse Curl	None	Negative	1	158
10	Circular Crunch	None	Basic Version	1	156
11	Pullover	Dumbbell	Basic Version	1	174
12	Lat Pulldown with Band	Exercise band	Basic Version	2	178
13	Chest Fly	Dumbbells	Pyramid	3	182
14	Shoulder Press plus Lateral Raise	Dumbbells	Superset	1	186, 188
15	Triceps Extension with Band	Exercise band	Negative	1	194
16	Seated Biceps Curl	Dumbbells	Negative	1	196

Gym Routines

The Buns of Steel Total-Body Workout is an excellent way to get in shape anywhere, anytime. The *Buns of Steel* videos are also great for the same reason. But perhaps you want to work out with a friend, try a new machine, or need the motivation of other people working out around you once in a while. That's the time to head for the nearest local health club or gym.

It's easy to adapt your toning routines from this book for the gym. You can bring your exercise equipment with you (step, exercise band, and so on) and look for a free area on the gym floor to do your usual Buns routine. Most clubs have good-quality equipment that does approximately the same movements you've been doing in your target toning workouts. If you decide to use the equipment, be sure to ask a qualified instructor for some guidance.

Note that not every exercise has a machine counterpart. You can double up on sets of something else if you can't find an equivalent machine. Or find a space where it isn't too crowded to do your normal target toning exercise.

HOT BODY TIP

Calorie basics: To figure out your basic calorie requirement, multiply your ideal weight by twelve. Your ideal weight is one that puts you at a healthy body fat percentage.

HOT BODY TIP

When doing an exercise, emphasize full range of motion. Think of every repetition as having a beginning, middle, and end. Concentrate on feeling your muscles work through all three points. If you do this correctly, you'll increase not only tone and strength, but flexibility as well.

BUNS OF STEEL EXERCISE	PAGE NUMBER	HEALTH CLUB MACHINE EQUIVALENT
Squat	60	Standing Squat; Leg Press; Hack Squat
Glute Raise or Kneeling Glute Raise with Band	78, 80	Glute Raise Machine
All Outer Thigh Exercises	92–99	Leg Abductor
All Inner Thigh Exercises	100–107	Leg Adductor
Standing Leg Extension with Band	122	Leg Extension
Bump Squat	124	Sissy Squat Station
Kneeling Four-Count Leg Curl	130	Leg Curl or Seated Leg Curl
Standing Leg Curl with Band	128	Standing Leg Curl
Standing Calf Raise off Step	132	Standing Calf Raise or Donkey Calf Raise
Seated Calf Raise	134	Seated Calf Raise
Basic Crunch, Total Crunch, Crunch and Pulse	148, 152, 154	Abdominal or Abdominal Crunch
Reverse Curl	158	Abdominal; Hip Flexion; High Chair; Roman Chair
Crossover Crunch, Circular Crunch	150, 156	Rotary Torso
Waist Bend with Band	162	Cable Waist Bend Exercises
Pullover	174	Pullover; Superpullover
Seated Row with Band	176	Seated Row; Low Row; Pulley Row; T-Bar Row
Lat Pulldown with Band	178	Lat Pulldown
Push-up	180	Bench Press; Smith Press; Decline Press; Chest Press
Chest Fly	182	Arm Cross; Butterfly; Pec Deck; Incline Fly
Shoulder Press	186	Shoulder Press

BUNS OF STEEL EXERCISE	PAGE NUMBER	HEALTH CLUB MACHINE EQUIVALENT
Lateral Raise	188	Lateral Raise
Upright Row with Band	190	Low Pulley
Triceps Extension with Band	194	Triceps Extension; Triceps Press; Dipping Station; Pushdown
Seated Biceps Curl	196	Biceps Curl; Preacher Curl
Standing Biceps Curl with Band	198	Low Pulley

HOT BODY TIP

Target toning not only makes you look terrific, it's a great confidence booster as well. Your newly reshaped body adds up to greater physical strength and stronger self-esteem.

HOT BODY TIP

Shake salt out of your diet. Too much sodium causes bloating and contributes to high blood pressure. The best way to reduce sodium intake: Pass up the salt shaker at the dinner table. Most Americans get more than enough sodium from the foods they eat without shaking on extra.

HOT BODY TIP

Most women lose 1 percent of their bone density each year after thirty. You can slow down bone loss by eating a diet that includes calcium-rich foods like skim milk, broccoli, and salmon (with the bones). Target toning also keeps bones healthy and strong.

Glossary

Advanced Exerciser. Someone who can perform the majority of the advanced versions of the target toning exercises and who can complete the twenty-minute isolation routines without undue strain. Usually this is someone who has been participating regularly in a target toning program for six months or more.

Aerobic. Sustained exercise such as walking, running, or cycling, which requires oxygen for fuel. Involves the repetitive, rhythmic movement of large muscle groups such as buns and thighs and causes an elevation in heart rate. The most efficient calorie- and fat-burning form of exercise.

Alignment. Refers to posture. **Natural alignment** is an ideal posture in which your head is centered between your shoulders, your shoulders are relaxed backward and downward, your chest and rib cage are lifted, your abdominals are pulled in toward your spine, your lower body is relaxed, and your weight is distributed evenly between both feet.

Anaerobic. Short bursts of exercise, usually lasting less than a minute, designed to increase the power, strength, and tone of a muscle. It relies on cellular enzymes for fuel rather than oxygen. Target toning is an example of anaerobic exercise.

Beginning Exerciser. Someone who finds the basic versions of most target toning exercises and the ten-minute isolation routines a challenge. Usually this is someone who has not been participating in a target toning program, has participated regularly for less than three months, or who has participated in a low-intensity exercise routine for a longer period of time.

Body Blaster Routine. A longer, more intense target toning routine for intermediate and advanced exercisers. Works the entire body and utilizes specialized techniques.

Body Fat Percentage. A method of determining how much of your weight is fat and how much is lean body tissue, or muscle. Optimal body fat percentages for women are between 16 and 26 percent; for men, 12 to 20 percent.

Body Weight. Your weight in pounds, usually taken on a scale. This is not a good determinant of fitness because it does not distinguish how much of your body composition is fat and how much is muscle.

Cardiovascular. Aerobic exercise that works the heart and lungs and, if done on a regular basis, increases endurance and the efficiency of oxygen use.

Contraction. When a muscle responds to a force by shortening, lengthening, or pushing against it without changing length. A contraction is experienced in the form of tension in the muscle being worked.

Cooldown. A period immediately following heavy exercise during which light activity such as slow walking and stretching is done in order gradually to slow your heart rate and breathing.

Definition. Degree of muscular development that shows through the skin because of a low amount of body fat. Having good definition is also known as being **muscular, cut, sculpted**, or **chiseled**.

Dumbbell. A short-handled weight bar used to add resistance to an exercise.

Ectomorph. A body type characterized by hips and shoulders approximately the same width, small to medium bones, and a lanky, angular appearance.

Endomorph. A body type characterized by hips wider than the shoulders, large bones, and a curvy, rounded appearance.

Exercise. Refers to the actual movement you are doing in a workout—for instance, a squat in a buns workout or a wall sit in a leg workout.

Exercise band or tube. A sturdy elastic band or tube (with or without handles) designed specifically for exercise. Some brand names include Dyna-band, Exer-tubing, and Spri. (Surgical tubing may be used as a suitable substitute.)

Fat Burner Circuit. A method of target toning that involves doing all of your exercises in quick succession with no rest in between.

Fitness. The ability to function optimally. **Fitness level** refers to your present level of physical condition.

Flexibility. Refers to the degree of mobility or the range of motion a joint can move through. A consistent program of stretching exercises increases flexibility.

Holds. A method of increasing intensity by holding an exercise at the top or bottom of a movement. An **isometric hold** increases the contraction duration of a muscle. In other instances, holding increases the amount of stretch you experience.

Intensity. The quality of effort you put into a workout or individual exercise.

Intermediate Exerciser. Someone who can easily complete the basic versions of most target toning exercises but cannot yet complete the more advanced versions without undue strain. The fifteen-minute isolation routines provide the most suitable workout for this individual. Usually this is someone who has been participating regularly in a target toning program for three to six months.

Interval Training. A type of workout routine where short periods of one type of exercise are interspersed with another. For instance, one minute of brisk walking is alternated with sets of target toning exercises. This is done to speed up the workout and to derive some of the benefits of both types of exercise (in other words, some aerobic benefits and some toning and strength benefits).

Isolation Routine. A target toning routine that focuses on one specific area of your body.

Locked. Refers to a joint such as the knee or elbow when it is fully extended, or "hyperextended." This puts undue pressure on the joint and throws off body alignment.

Mesomorph. A body type characterized by shoulders slightly wider than the hips, medium to large bones, and a muscular, athletic appearance.

Mind/Body Focus. Something that helps link your thought process with your body's movement. Often this is done by relating the movement to something that is familiar.

Negatives. A Body Blaster technique in which you give equal time to both the lifting and lowering phases of an exercise.

Program. An entire exercise schedule, as in the Buns of Steel Total-Body Workout program.

Pulses. A method of increasing the intensity of an exercise by bringing the arm or leg to the top of the movement and then lifting and lowering it a very small distance, usually no more than one or two inches in either direction. This puts continuous tension on the muscle by forcing it to sustain a contraction.

Pyramids. A Body Blaster technique that involves making each set of an exercise progressively harder. Usually this is done by adding slightly more weight with each new set. In **descending pyramids**, the weight gets progressively lighter with each set.

Radial artery. A point on the side of your wrist directly below your thumb where your pulse is located.

Rated Perceived Exertion (RPE). A method of measuring intensity that utilizes a scale to relate your perception of the difficulty to the physical effort of the exercise.

Repetition (rep or reps). A complete movement of an exercise.

Rest. The briefest possible interval between sets that allows the working muscle to regain full strength. Also: the time interval between workouts.

Routine. A group of exercises.

Set. A group of continuously performed repetitions. In target toning a set consists of eight to fifteen repetitions.

Soft. Not fully straightened, as it applies to a joint such as the knee or elbow.

Split Routine. A method of training in which different muscle groups are target toned on different days.

Spot reducing. An ineffective method of training that involves performing a high number of repetitions at a low intensity.

Step. A platform used to add height to an exercise. Usually consists of a platform with a rubberized, nonslip platform and one or more sets of **risers**, which are used to increase the step's elevation.

Supercircuit. A method of training where a brief interval of an aerobic activity is alternated with a set of target toning with no rest period in between. A type of **interval** training.

Superset. A Body Blaster technique that involves combining two sets of two different exercises with no rest in between.

Talk Test. A method of determining aerobic exercise intensity where you gauge the difficulty of talking as you exercise.

Target Heart Rate Range. The number of times your heart beats per minute in the range that keeps you exercising aerobically at the appropriate intensity level. The most common method of determining this is with the **age predicted formula**: subtract your age from 220 and then multiply it by 60 and 85 percent (or .60 and .85).

Target Toning. A method of training that utilizes resistance and precise, focused movements to bring about increases in tone, definition, and muscular strength.

Training Range. The minimum and the maximum workout intensity for safe and effective exercise.

Warm-up. The period of time where you engage in light activities such as walking or easy jogging in order to prepare your body for hard physical exercise. The warm-up period increases the blood flow to your muscles, speeds up heart rate, and elevates body temperature.

Whole-Body Training. A method of training in which you train your entire body with a single routine rather than a series of isolation routines.

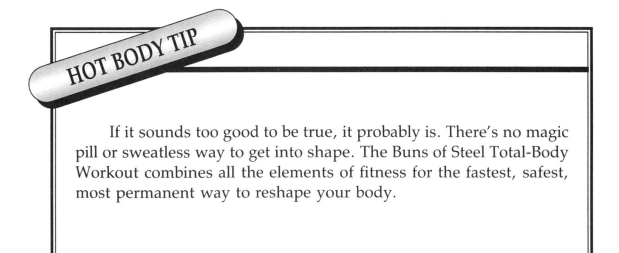

HOT BODY TIP

If it sounds too good to be true, it probably is. There's no magic pill or sweatless way to get into shape. The Buns of Steel Total-Body Workout combines all the elements of fitness for the fastest, safest, most permanent way to reshape your body.

Afterword

Now that you've read through the entire program, you know what it takes to make a success of your workout program. You also know that target toning is simply the best method of body shaping there is. Now it's time to put all that knowledge to good use!

You'll find that it's easy to stay motivated on the Buns of Steel Total-Body Workout program. For one thing, you'll be amazed at how quickly your body responds to target toning. You should see noticeable results after a few weeks of training—perhaps after the first couple of sessions. Just imagining the results should be enough to keep you coming back for more. Even if you don't have trouble zones per se, you'll still make visible improvements.

Another advantage to the Buns of Steel Total-Body Workout is how flexible it is. You're not locked into one routine. It's so easy to adapt the information in this book. You'll refer to it a lot in the beginning, but once you've learned proper exercise form and memorized your favorite exercise routines, you may not look at it quite as often. Does that mean you should stick this book in your bookshelf and forget about it? Of course not!

Even if you're happy to stay with the basics, you'll still need a refresher course from time to time. The basics may be fine for a while, but as you get firmer, more sculpted, and stronger, you'll want more of a challenge. That's the time to check out the exercise variations and the special routines. They'll provide you with infinite ways to restructure your program so it's always fresh and effective. In fact, think of the Buns of Steel Total-Body Workout as your personal target toning encyclopedia. You can refer to it any time you have a question or want to make a change in your exercise routine.

And don't forget the convenience of the Buns of Steel Total-Body Workout program. It's completely portable, so you can squeeze in a target toning session even if you're miles away from the nearest gym or VCR. Only have a few minutes? You can do an effective target toning routine in as little as five minutes. The Total-Body Workout makes it possible for you to work out anytime, anywhere.

The most important message we hope you take with you is that *anyone* can create a better body with the Buns of Steel target toning method. It doesn't matter where you're starting from. You can get to where you want to go. Just follow the exercise program we've detailed for you. It's that simple.

Good luck! Go for it!

INDEX

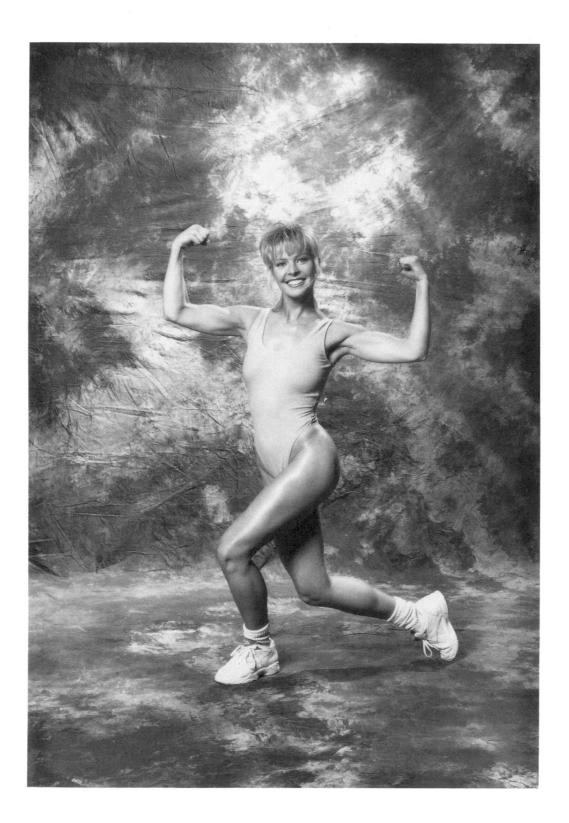

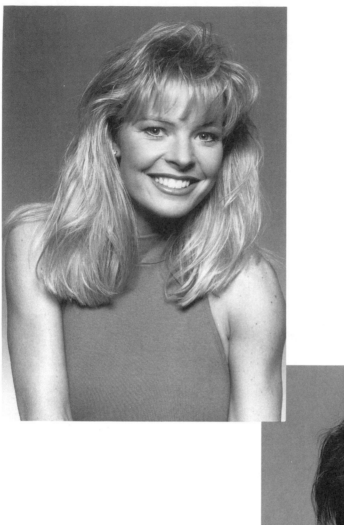

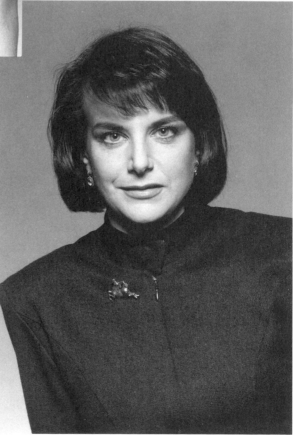

About the Authors

Leisa Hart is certified by The Health Instructor's Network (THIN) and the American Council on Exercise (ACE). She has ten years experience in the fitness industry as a personal trainer, competitor in professional fitness competitions, and sportscaster. Among her many accomplishments, she was first runner-up in the 1992 Fitness America Pageant and is a former reporter for *Sunday Night Show Time* and *This Week in the South West Conference*. Leisa, the daughter of a retired mechanical engineer and homemaker, is the youngest of ten children. She currently lives in Dallas, Texas.

Liz Neporent has a master's degree in exercise physiology and is certified by the American College of Sports Medicine (ACSM), ACE, and the National Strength and Conditioning Association (NSCA). She is president of Frontline Fitness, a New York-based fitness consulting company. She is a contributing editor at *Longevity* magazine and *Women's Sports and Fitness* magazine and is a frequent contributor to *Shape, Self, Men's Fitness, Family Circle*, and others. The daughter of a physician and travel agent, Liz currently resides in New York City with her husband, Jay Shafran.

TRY THE LATEST **VIDEOS** FROM
BUNS OF STEEL

Need to concentrate on firming a specific part of your body or just want to relieve stress? BUNS OF STEEL has a video right for YOU! BUNS OF STEEL helps you get the body you've always wanted.

BUNS OF STEEL SERIES
Target toning exercise programs that get results!

- BUNS OF STEEL: The Original

- BUNS OF STEEL 2: Beginners Step

- BUNS OF STEEL 3: Buns and More!

- BUNS OF STEEL 4: Advanced Workout

- BUNS OF STEEL 5: Beginners Workout

- BUNS OF STEEL 6: Intermediate Step

- BUNS OF STEEL 7: Advanced Step

- BUNS OF STEEL 8: Pregnancy Workout

- BUNS OF STEEL 9: Post Pregnancy

- ABS OF STEEL

- ABS OF STEEL 2: Advanced

- ARMS AND ABS OF STEEL

- LEGS OF STEEL

- THIGHS OF STEEL

BUNS OF STEEL PLATINUM SERIES
All the great benefits of target toning plus aerobics for weight loss!

- BUNS OF STEEL 2000

- ABS OF STEEL 2000

- THIGHS OF STEEL 2000

- ARMS AND ABS OF STEEL 2000

- BUNS OF STEEL STEP 2000

- LEGS OF STEEL 2000

- ABS AND CHEST OF STEEL 2000

MEN OF STEEL SERIES
A series designed exclusively by men, for men!

- ABS OF STEEL FOR MEN

- ARMS OF STEEL FOR MEN

- LEGS OF STEEL FOR MEN

MIND/BODY SERIES
Great for relieving stress and improving flexibility.

- BUNS OF STEEL TAI CHI

- BUNS OF STEEL YOGA

AVAILABLE AT YOUR LOCAL VIDEO AND SPORTING GOODS STORES!